TOILET TRAINING

from the Inside Out

When connection matters more than doing it "right"

ELISE HANSFORD

CONTENTS

INTRODUCTION

WHY THIS BOOK EXISTS

T oilet training is one of those milestones everyone talks about — but barely anyone talks about the emotional reality of it.

The holding.

The accidents.

The fear.

The pressure.

The overwhelm.

The comparison.

The moments you question yourself.

The tears — yours and theirs.

The quiet moments when you sit on the floor afterward and wonder,
"Am I doing this right?"

Most books focus on timelines, steps, readiness checklists, and outcomes. Very few talk about the nervous system, emotional safety, connection, or the internal world a child must feel before their body can truly let go.

Very few books speak to the parent's experience — the exhaustion, the doubt, the loneliness, the emotional load that sits on your shoulders as you try to guide a tiny human through something so big.

And that is why this book exists.

This book is here to support you in the midst of toilet learning — the uncertainty, the waiting, the doubt, the days that don't look like progress.

The outcome does not come from following the steps perfectly. It comes from your child, in their own time.

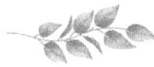

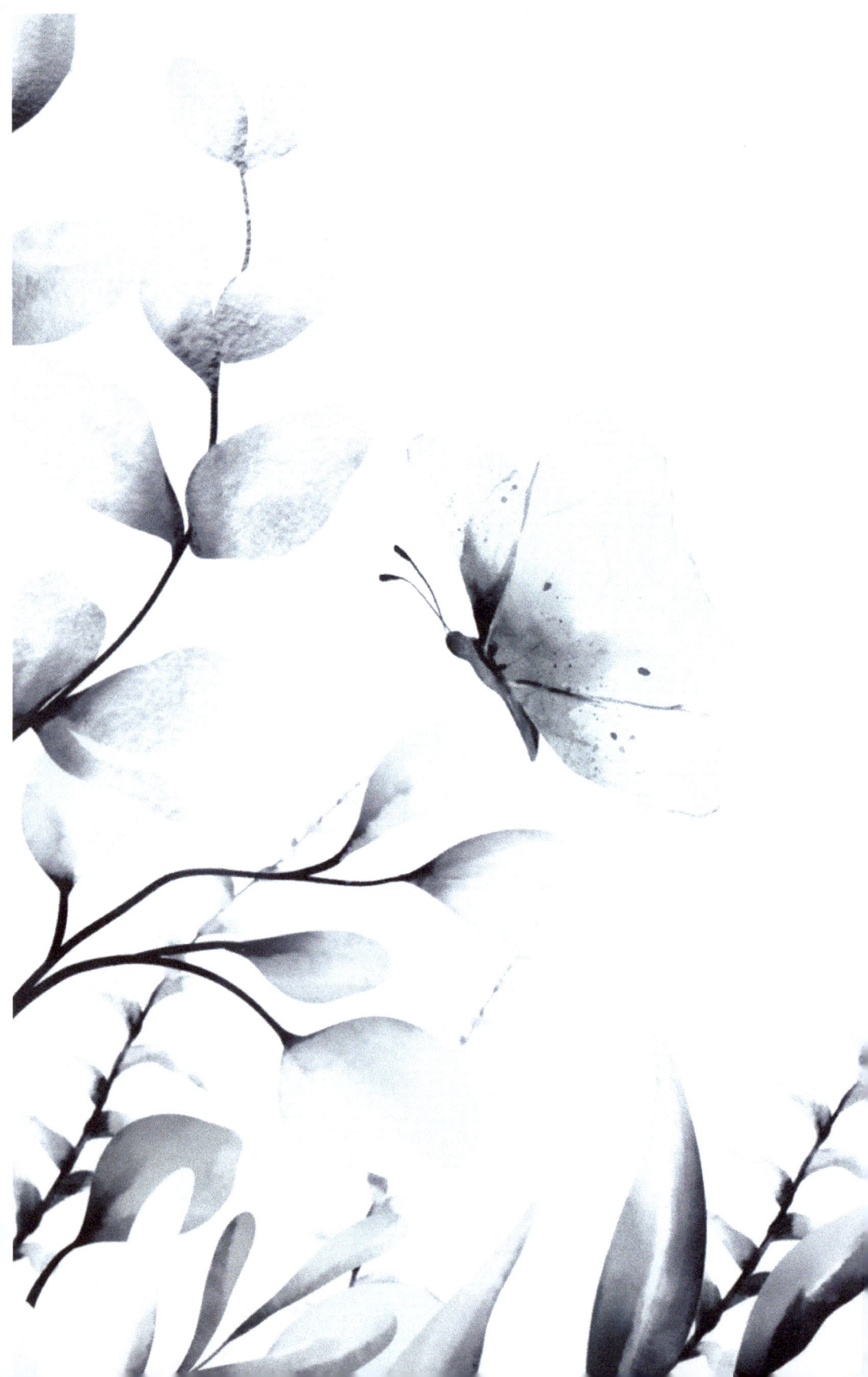

A Little About Me, and Why I'm Writing This

I'm not a professional toilet-training expert. I'm a mum of three — just like many of you reading this.

I've walked this path three different times, with three different children, and each experience has unfolded in its own way.

My journey with my middle child, Charlie, unfolded differently again.

Not wrong.
Not broken.
Just different.

She taught me to slow down, to listen more closely, and to understand toilet learning from the inside out

— through her body, her emotions, and her nervous system.

This book grew from that learning.

I'm a mum who has cried on the bathroom floor.
A mum who has wiped tears — theirs and mine.
A mum who has Googled things at 2am.
A mum who has tried, paused, reset, and tried again.

A mum who needed a book like this long before I ever wrote it.

Along the way, I realised something important.

Toilet learning isn't just a skill.

It's a relationship.
It's nervous-system work.
It's emotional safety.
It's connection.
It's trust.
It's learning to understand your child in ways you maybe never had to before.

This book is written from that place — the lived place, not the clinical one.

It's written for parents who feel overwhelmed, unseen, or unsure.

Parents who don't have a village.

Parents doing this with multiple children.

Parents navigating neurodivergence, late-talking, sensory needs, and emotional dysregulation.

Parents who feel like they're failing, when really, they're showing extraordinary love.

This is a book for real families — not perfect ones.

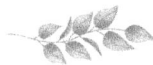

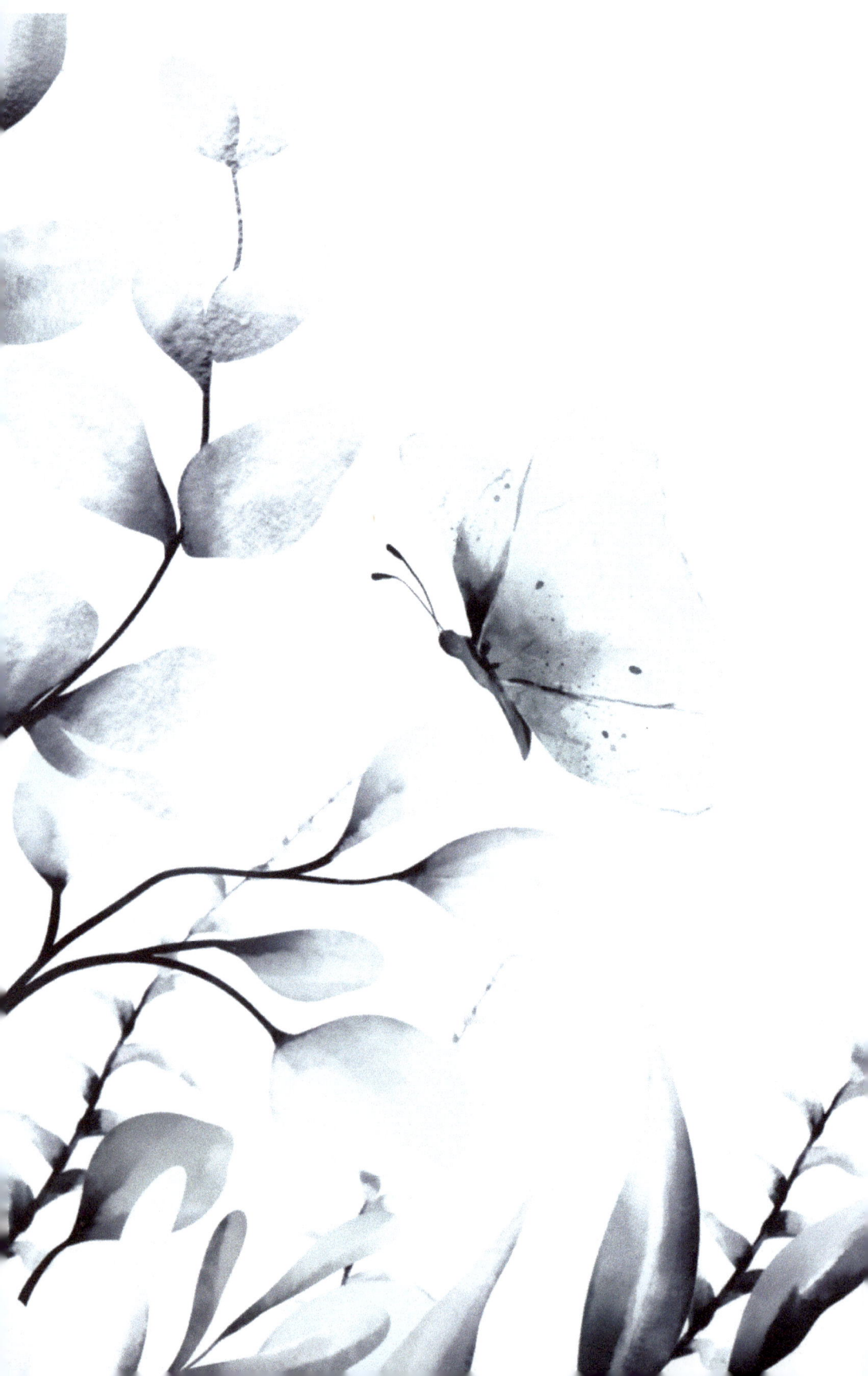

WHAT THIS BOOK IS — AND WHAT IT ISN'T

This is not a race to underwear.
This is not about forcing readiness.
This is not about quick results.
This is not about doing it "right."

This is about:

- connection before correction

- safety before skill

- regulation before release

- trust before independence

- understanding before achievement

Because toilet learning doesn't start when the nappy comes off.

It starts when your child feels safe enough to try.
It starts when *you* feel supported enough to guide them.

This is toilet learning from the inside out.

And you don't have to walk it alone.

 I'm right here — walking it with you.

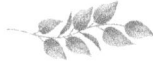

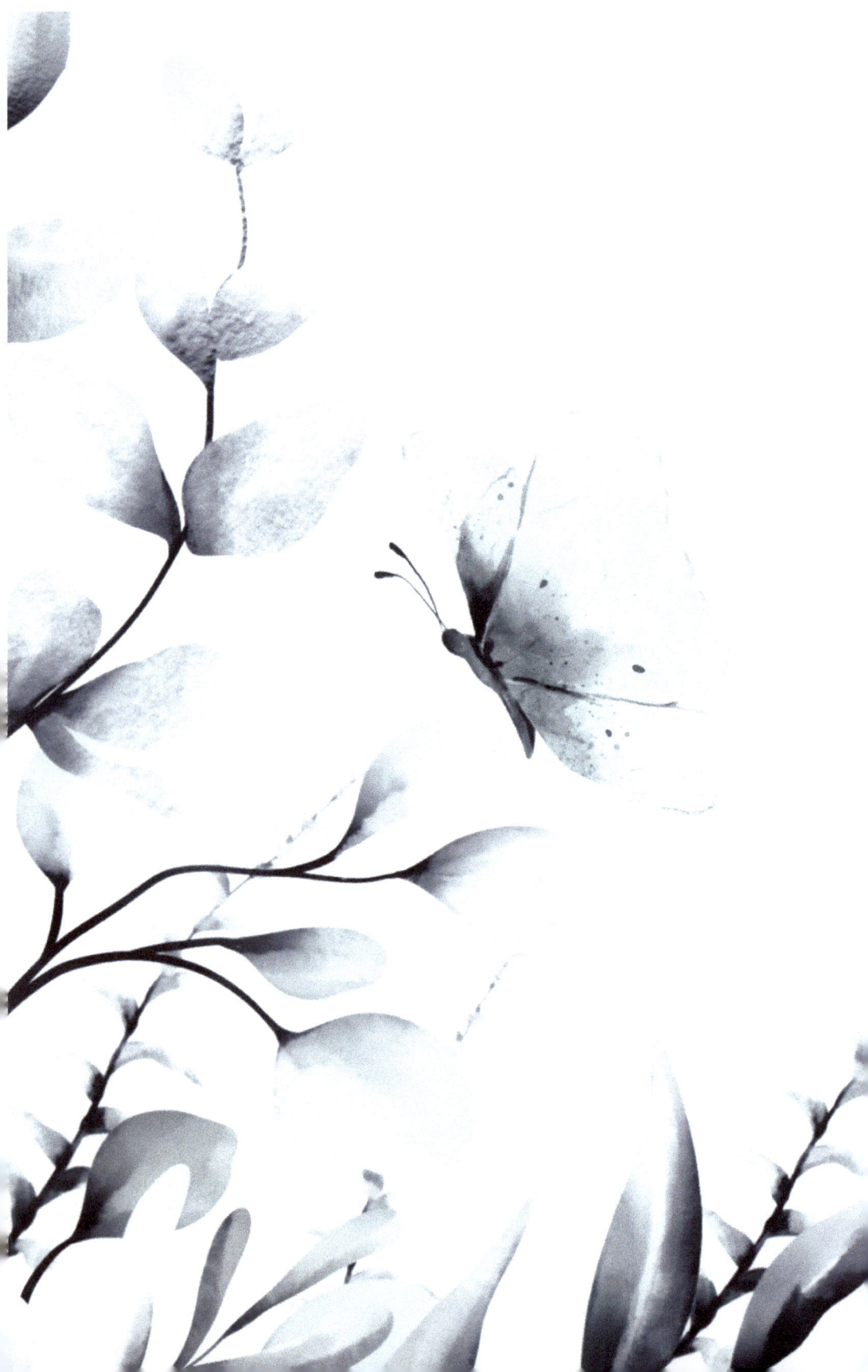

AUTHOR'S NOTE

This book was written quietly, in the in-between moments of motherhood.

Between snack requests and school drop-offs.
Between sleepless nights and early mornings.
Between wiping floors, holding little bodies, and holding myself together.

I wrote this as a mum — not an expert, not a clinician — but as someone deeply inside it.

I'm a mother of three, living in Australia, raising my children in the real rhythm of family life — where days don't always go to plan, where support can feel far away, and where the mental load of mothering is often invisible.

There were moments early on when I cried for days — not because of accidents, but because I truly believed I was failing my child.

I didn't need another method.
I needed reassurance.
I needed permission to slow down and listen — to my child, and to myself.

This book comes from lived experience.

From sitting on the bathroom floor after accidents.
From pausing a process that felt too much.
From learning — sometimes the hard way — that children don't release when they feel watched, rushed, or pressured.

They release when they feel safe.

I wrote this for the parent reading at night after everyone else is asleep.
For the one wondering why this feels harder than they

were told.

For the one comparing their child to others and quietly blaming themselves.

For the one navigating sensitive temperaments, late communication, big emotions, or neurodivergent needs.

You won't find perfection in these pages.
You'll find permission.

Permission to slow down.
Permission to listen.
Permission to trust your child — and yourself.

This book doesn't ask you to override your instincts.
It asks you to come back to them.

If, as you read, you feel seen —
If your shoulders soften a little —
If you realise you're not failing, you're responding —
then this book has done what it was meant to do.

You are not behind.
Your child is not broken.
And you are not alone.

With deep respect for the work you're doing,

Elise Hansford

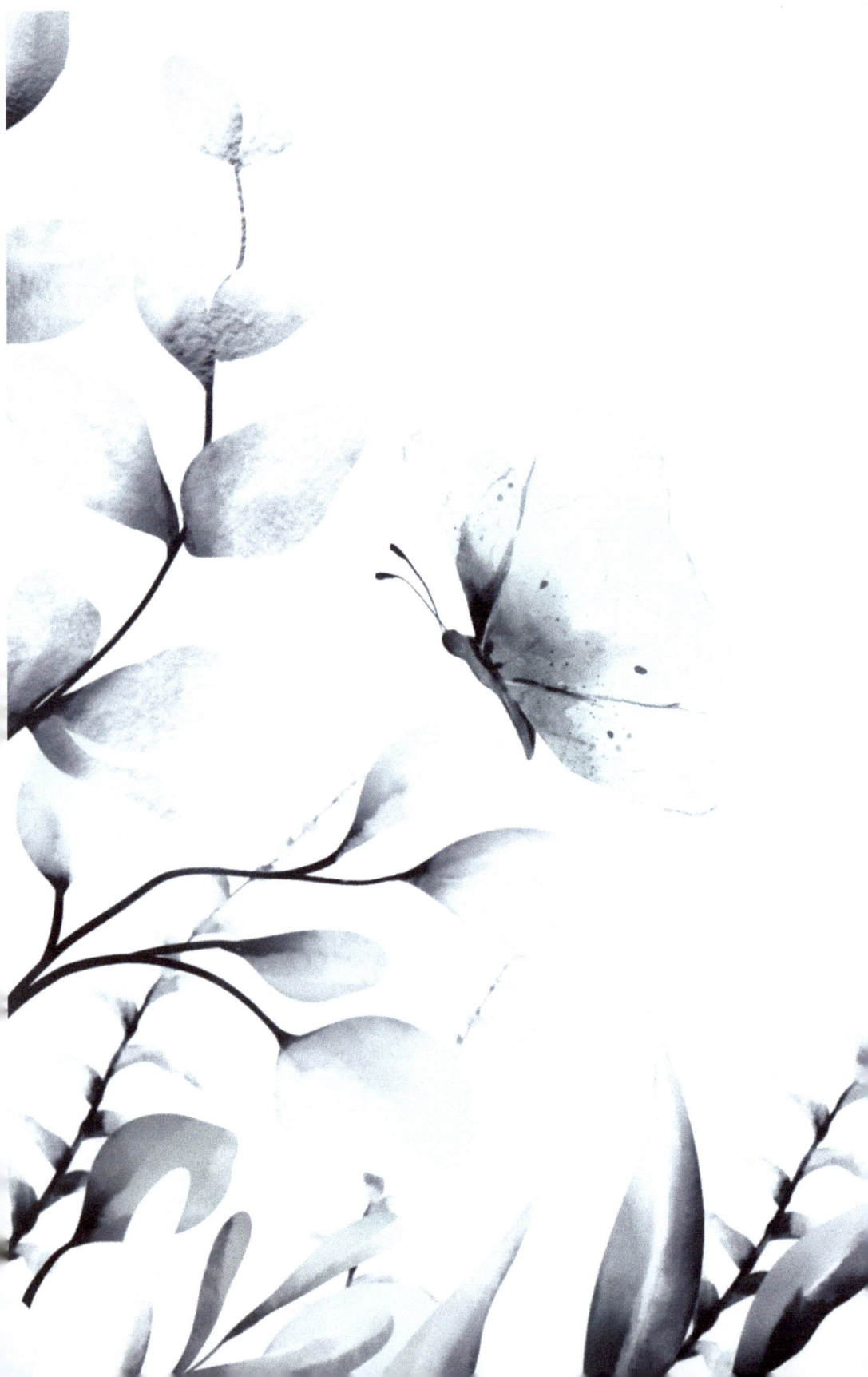

CHAPTER 1

The Parent's Emotional Journey

Before we talk about toilets, potties, timing, or techniques...

Hi. I'm really glad you're here.

Take a breath.

You don't have to have it all figured out to be here.

This part of the journey isn't just about your child — it's about you as well. And you deserve to be seen in it.

Toilet learning is not just a developmental milestone for children. It is an emotional journey for parents too. Often a quiet one. An invisible one. One that unfolds mostly inside your body and your mind, long before anything changes in the toilet.

It's a journey filled with hope and doubt living side by side. With moments of confidence that quickly give way to uncertainty. With pride in your child, followed closely by fear that you're getting something wrong.

It's the pressure you feel when progress doesn't look the way you expected. The comparison that sneaks in when other children seem to "just get it." The frustration you don't want to admit out loud. And the deep, aching love that makes you care so much it hurts.

Sometimes all in the same day.
Sometimes all in the same moment.

And yet, so few guides pause here. So few stop to say: this is hard for parents too.

Most resources focus on what your child should do — but barely touch on what you carry while supporting them. This part often goes unseen.

But here, it doesn't.

The Quiet Pressure Parents Carry

At some point, many parents begin to feel it.

An unspoken countdown.

A sense that time is ticking — even if no one says it out loud.

Questions start to creep in, often in the quiet moments:

Should my child be doing this by now?
Why does it seem so easy for other families?
Am I doing something wrong?
What if we've missed the window?

This pressure rarely arrives loudly.

It shows up in passing comments. In milestone charts. In watching other children move ahead. In the way your body tightens when the topic comes up.

Sometimes the pressure comes from outside — childcare expectations, family opinions, social media, well-meaning advice that lands heavier than intended.

And sometimes it comes from inside — from your own hopes, fears, and the picture you once held of how this stage would unfold.

For parents of sensitive children, late talkers, neurodivergent children, or children who simply need more space and time, this pressure can feel especially heavy.

Because you may already be carrying years of:

• advocating when something didn't quite fit
• explaining your child to others
• waiting while peers moved ahead
• trusting your instincts while being told to hurry

So when toilet learning begins, it doesn't arrive on a clean slate.

It taps into old worries. Old comparisons. Old moments of doubt you thought you'd already worked through.

The pressure can build quietly — until even gentle decisions feel loaded.

So let this be said clearly:

You are allowed to slow this down.

You are allowed to pause.

You are allowed to choose softness over urgency.

You have not missed anything.

And your child's pace is not a problem to fix

When It Doesn't Look Like the "Three-Day Method"

Many parents come into toilet learning expecting momentum.

A quick shift. A clear before and after. A sense that once you start, you're meant to keep moving forward.

So when progress looks slow, uneven, or stop–start, it's easy to internalise it.

You might feel:

• disappointed, even when you know your child is trying

- worried when interest fades
- discouraged by accidents
- unsure whether to push forward or gently pull back

And beneath all of that, there's often a deeper fear:

What if this means something is wrong?

That fear makes sense.

It comes from caring deeply. From wanting to protect your child. From wanting to do right by them.

But toilet learning is not a test.

It is not a reflection of your parenting.

And it is not a measure of your child's intelligence, readiness, or future independence.

And it is okay that it doesn't look like the "three-day method."

Many children do not learn in straight lines.

Many need pauses, resets, or time for their bodies to catch up.

Needing more time does not mean failure.

It means learning is still happening — just quietly.

And quiet learning still counts.

The Exhaustion No One Warns You About

This is a tired that lives deeper than your muscles.

It settles into your nervous system. It hums beneath your day. It doesn't disappear with sleep.

It's the tired of being on all the time — watching cues, listening for silence, scanning for accidents, second-guessing every decision.

It's the tired of holding your child's emotions and your own — often at the same time.

Of staying calm on the outside while everything inside feels stretched thin.

You might find yourself:

• emotionally depleted by mid-morning
• crying in the laundry, the bathroom, or the car

- snapping — and then drowning in guilt
- lying awake replaying the day

Even when nothing "went wrong."

Especially when nothing makes sense yet.

This kind of exhaustion isn't about effort.

It's about constant emotional presence.

So if this is you — pause.

Drink the water.
Eat the food.
Sit down when you can.

Because you matter in this too.

And caring for yourself is not a distraction from this process — it's part of how you keep going.

The Invisible Weight Parents Carry

Toilet learning adds a layer of invisible labour that rarely gets named.

You are tracking progress that can't be measured.
Holding hope while managing disappointment.
Staying calm so your child can feel safe.
Carrying responsibility for an outcome you can't control.

You are thinking ahead. Replaying moments. Adjusting your approach. Holding it together quietly — even when you feel unsure.

Often while still caring for other children. Working. Running a household. Or healing parts of yourself that are already tired.

This work is constant, and it is unseen.

There is no finish-line applause.
No clear reassurance.
No moment where someone officially tells you, "You're doing enough."

Just the steady weight of responsibility — day after day.

And yet, you keep showing up.

That matters.

When You're Carrying It Mostly By Yourself

Many parents move through this stage without a true village.

For some, that means doing this without a partner at all.

For others, it means having people around — but still feeling alone in it.

So you carry it.

The decisions.
The wondering.
The quiet self-questioning.

You carry it in your body.
In your chest.
In the still moments when no one sees how hard you're trying.

For single parents, this weight can feel relentless.

There is no handover.
No shared mental load.
No break from being the one who holds it all.

If this is you, let this be said clearly:

You are not failing because this feels hard.

You are doing something profoundly demanding — often without enough support.

And you deserve to be seen here.

Holding Space for Mixed Emotions (and Nervous Systems)

It is possible to feel proud and exhausted.
Hopeful and overwhelmed.
Confident one moment and deeply uncertain the next.

This doesn't mean you're failing.

It means you're human.

There is no perfect emotional response.

Only honest ones.

If toilet learning has begun to feel tense or emotionally charged, it doesn't mean you need to try harder.

Often, it means something needs softening.

Pressure — even quiet, loving pressure — is felt by the body.

Both yours.
And your child's.

Letting Go of Comparison

Every child's body learns in its own time.

Every family's journey looks different.

And yes — it is okay if your child takes more time.

Taking longer does not mean something is wrong.

It does not mean your child is behind.

It simply means this is their pace.

Different does not mean wrong.

And Then — Slowly — Something Shifts

For most families, there comes a moment.

Not dramatic.

Not perfect.

But real.

A small win feels huge.

Hope flickers.

And suddenly, the path forward feels possible.

A Gentle Send-Off

Before you turn the page — pause.

Take another breath.

You are allowed to slow this down.

You are allowed to trust yourself.

And you are already doing more right than you realise.

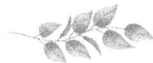

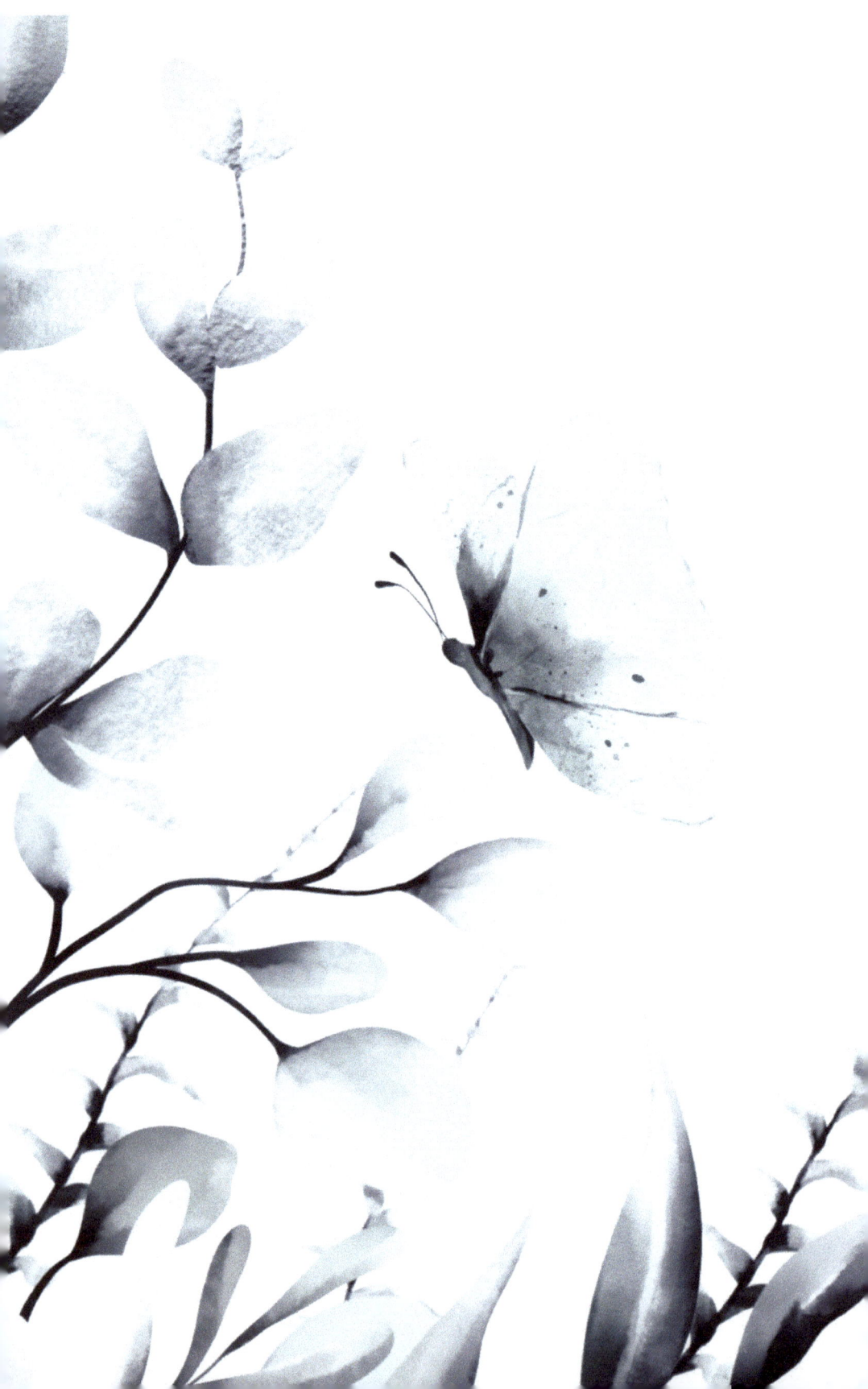

CHAPTER 2

Understanding Your Child

B efore we talk about readiness signs, routines, or toilets themselves, we need to pause here. Take a moment. Because toilet learning doesn't begin in the bathroom. It doesn't begin with a potty, a seat, or a schedule. It begins inside your child.

Every child arrives at toilet learning carrying a completely unique inner world — a different nervous system, a different pace, a different relationship with their body, and a different way of meeting change. Some children move toward new experiences with curiosity. Others need time to watch, feel, and trust first. Some notice every sensation in their body. Others are still learning how to hear those signals at all.

None of these differences mean anything is wrong. They are not flaws to fix. They are not delays to push through. They are simply signs that your child is human — learning in the only way their body and brain know how.

And when we start from that understanding, everything else becomes gentler.

Seeing Your Child Beyond the Checklist

Many parents are offered lists:

• Can they pull their pants down?
• Can they sit still?
• Do they follow instructions?
• Do they show interest?

These lists are usually shared with good intentions. But they can quietly create pressure — and doubt — where there doesn't need to be any.

Children are not checkboxes. They are not behind. They are not failing just because their journey unfolds differently.

If this feels heavy to read, it's because you care — and that care already matters more than any checklist.

Some children seem capable on the outside but feel unsure on the inside. Others appear uninterested while their nervous system is still finding its footing.

You might recognise moments like:

• A child sitting on the toilet, chatting comfortably, but nothing happening
• A child realising they're weeing only once it has already started
• A child who talks confidently about using the toilet, yet feels hesitant when it's time

These moments aren't mistakes. They're messages. They show us how a child is experiencing learning — where they feel safe, where they feel unsure, and what they may need more time with.

Understanding a child isn't about pushing them forward. It's about staying close enough to notice what they're telling us.

<u>Different Inner Worlds, Different Needs</u>

Every child brings their own inner world into toilet learning.

Some children feel things deeply. They notice change. They take time to trust what's being asked of them. These children often like to watch first. To take things in slowly. To feel settled before they try.

You might notice a child who:

• Needs time before sitting or attempting
• Pulls back when they feel watched or hurried
• Becomes quiet or resistant when expectations suddenly increase

What helps these children most isn't pressure or encouragement to push through — it's reassurance, patience, and knowing there's no rush.

Other children experience the world through movement and action. Their bodies lead the way. They're curious, busy, and deeply absorbed in what they're doing.

You might notice a child who:

• Only realises they need to go at the very last moment
• Wees while standing, squatting, or mid-play
• Finds it hard to stop what they're doing to sit

What helps these children most isn't correction or discipline — it's gentle support noticing their body and making sense of those signals.

Neither way of being is easier. Neither is harder. They are simply different ways of moving through the world.

When toilet learning follows a child's inner world — rather than trying to reshape it — things tend to soften. Children feel understood instead of managed. And learning is given the space it needs to unfold.

Body Awareness Comes Before Control

One of the hardest parts of toilet learning — and one of the most misunderstood — is what's happening inside a child's body.

Before a child can use the toilet, their body has to learn something new. It has to notice a sensation. Make sense of it. And trust that it's safe to respond.

For many children, this doesn't happen all at once.

Some children are still learning how their body speaks to them. Some feel the signal suddenly, like a rush. Some feel it too late. And some feel it clearly, but freeze when the moment arrives.

You might recognise this in moments like:

• A child weeing on the floor and announcing "I'm weeing" as it's happening
• A child telling you they need to go only once it's already over
• A child holding on until they're visibly uncomfortable
• A child who wants independence, yet resists sitting

These moments can be confusing — and sometimes frustrating. If this is where your child is right now, it doesn't mean you've missed a window or done something wrong.

They aren't acts of defiance. They aren't refusal. They are signs of a body still learning its own language.

When we slow down enough to listen to what the body is doing, we stop pushing for control — and start supporting awareness. And awareness is where learning begins.

Different Brains, Same Need for Safety

Every child's brain takes in the world a little differently.

Some notice everything. Some feel change deeply. Some experience the world in ways that others don't always see.

Other children move through change more easily. They adapt quickly. They seem less affected by noise, clothing, or transitions — and some even appear to thrive when gentle expectations are introduced.

Both experiences are real. Both are valid.

Different brains don't change what children need —
they change how strongly those needs are felt, and how
they show up.

Sensitivity, confidence, and curiosity all sit side by side
on a wide, human spectrum.

What helps all children is:

• Predictability, so their body knows what's coming
• Choice, so they feel a sense of control
• Emotional reassurance, so mistakes don't feel unsafe
• Low-pressure opportunities to try, without
expectation

When children feel safe, their nervous systems soften.
When their nervous systems soften, their bodies are
more able to release. And when the body feels safe,
learning becomes possible again.

Meeting a child where they are — instead of where we
think they should be — is often the moment progress
gently returns.

When Learning Starts to Feel Like Too Much

Toilet learning asks a lot of a small body. It asks a child to notice something unfamiliar, to pause what they're doing, and to let go — all while staying calm enough to feel safe.

Sometimes, without anyone meaning to, learning begins to feel watched. Or rushed. Or quietly measured.

And when that happens, a child's body may begin to protect itself. Muscles tighten. Awareness narrows. Signals that once felt clear become harder to find.

This is often when parents notice a shift — progress followed by resistance, or a child who can only go when no one is watching.

These moments aren't stubbornness. They're not a step backwards. They're the body saying, "This feels like too much right now."

And when a body feels overwhelmed, protection always comes before progress.

Where Readiness Really Lives

We're often told readiness is something to look for. An age. A skill. A sign that says, *now*.

And while those signs can be helpful, they're often misunderstood. Because for many children, readiness doesn't suddenly appear — it's something that's been quietly building long before anyone decides to try.

Before a child ever sits on the toilet, they're already doing important work. They're learning about their body. They're watching how things work. They're taking in your language, your tone, your reactions.

So when readiness signs do show up — interest, awareness, staying dry for longer — they aren't the beginning. They're the result.

For Charlie, readiness didn't arrive as a big moment or a clear milestone. It showed up quietly. She began asking to sit on the big toilet — my toilet — just like I did. She followed me into the bathroom. She watched. She was curious.

There was no pressure. No expectation that anything had to happen.

But together, those small signs told me something important: her interest was growing, and her sense of safety in that space already existed. That's when we knew it was time to gently begin.

For many children, readiness isn't something they perform. It's something they feel.

Readiness lives in trust. In knowing they're safe with you. In feeling allowed to try — and allowed to stop. In being accepted, even when nothing happens.

Sometimes progress looks quiet:

• Sitting and chatting
• Trying and stopping
• Saying "not today"
• Staying dry a little longer

These moments are not wasted. They are building safety. And safety is what learning grows from.

You Know Your Child Best

You live with your child. You see the tiny shifts others don't notice. The hesitation before trying. The moments when their body tightens — and when it softens again.

You know when something feels off. And when something feels right.

Nothing is wrong with your child. Nothing is broken. Nothing has been missed.

When you understand your child, the questions change.

Instead of asking, *"Why aren't they doing this yet?"*

You begin to ask, *"What does my child need to feel safe enough to learn?"*

That question softens everything. It builds trust. And it changes the journey — for both of you.

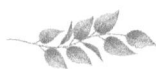

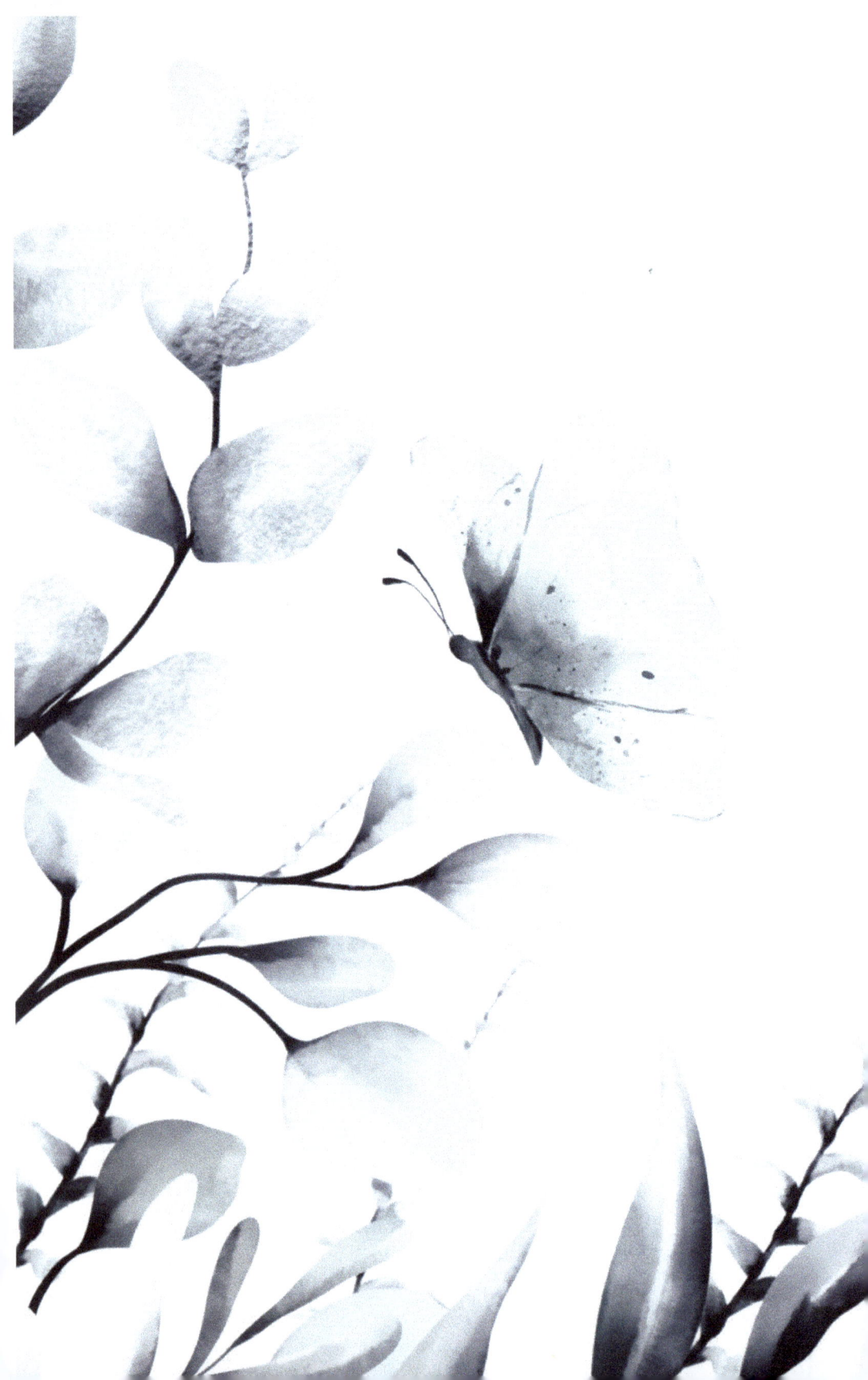

CHAPTER 3

Creating a Safe, Supportive Environment

B efore a child ever releases on the toilet, they need to feel emotionally and physically safe.

It begins with how your child feels — in their body, in their home, and especially in their relationship with you. A space where their body can soften enough to try, where they feel supported enough to trust the process, and connected enough to let go.

This chapter brings together the practical and the heart-led, showing how safety — not pressure — is what allows learning to unfold.

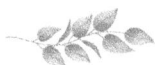

1. Learning Begins With Seeing

One of the most powerful teaching tools your child has is simply you.

Many children become interested in the toilet simply by watching. Not through lessons. Not through pressure. Through curiosity.

When children see us use the toilet calmly and confidently, they absorb that experience. They are not just watching what we do — they are sensing how it feels.

Leaving the door open.
Inviting your child in.
Letting them watch without pressure.

All of this builds familiarity around toileting.

Children learn through:

• watching

• sensing

• listening

• being near your calm presence

They don't need a demonstration video.
They need you.

Charlie learned more from watching me than from any book or routine. She saw safety. She saw normality. She saw that nothing scary was happening.

When toileting is open and unforced, safety forms quietly — and from that safety, progress follows.

2. Preparing the Environment

Bathrooms can be overwhelming for young children — echoey, cold, unpredictable, and loud.

Some children fear the toilet not because they "don't want to," but because their nervous system feels unsure.

Your bathroom setup quietly teaches your child what to expect here. Whether this is a place of safety. Whether their body can relax. Whether they can trust themselves in this space.

The environment invites learning.
It never enforces it.

When the space feels safe, the body follows.

Toilet, Potty, or Both

There is no single "right" option.

Some children feel more secure closer to the ground.
Some children prefer the big toilet.
Some move between both.

What matters most is that your child feels stable and supported.

If a child feels frightened by a training ladder or the height of the big toilet, a simple seat insert with a sturdy step stool can feel much safer.

Follow your child's comfort — not the product label.

3. A Supportive Toilet Setup

A supportive toilet setup helps a child's body feel grounded and secure.

When a child feels physically stable, their nervous system has less work to do — and relaxation becomes possible.

This doesn't require a perfect setup or special equipment. It simply means paying attention to how your child's body responds.

Supportive setups often include:

• a secure seat insert or stable ladder
• feet that are fully supported
• soft, comfortable lighting
• a sturdy step stool
• a comfortable potty placed in a calm, familiar spot

Charlie once struggled deeply with a ladder-style seat. It felt high, unstable, and unpredictable to her body.

When I switched to a simple seat insert and a sturdy stool, her whole body softened. She could settle. She could stay.

The right setup doesn't shout instructions.
It quietly reassures.

It whispers: *"You're safe here. You can trust this place."*

4. Sensory Support: Toys and Comfort Items

Some toddlers — especially sensitive, neurodivergent, late-talking children, or those who don't thrive under pressure — need more than a routine to feel safe.

They may need sensory support.

A toy.
A book.
An iPad.
A sensory fidget.
A favourite song.

These are not distractions.
They are anchors.

To a child, holding something familiar sends a powerful message:

- "I'm safe."
- "This feels okay."
- "I can stay here."

Comfort items help regulate the nervous system. They can reduce fear, ease uncertainty, and support a child to remain seated long enough for their body to respond.

For some children, these supports bridge the gap between discomfort and trust.

Screens and toys do not prevent learning.
They make learning possible.

A regulated child can listen to their body.
A dysregulated child is focused on protection.

Regulation comes first.
Learning follows.

5. Gentle Choices Build Confidence

Choices reduce resistance because they give children a sense of ownership.

Toilet learning can feel vulnerable. Children don't always understand what is being asked of them, or why their body suddenly feels different.

Choice softens that vulnerability. It helps a child feel included rather than directed, supported rather than pushed.

Gentle choices might look like:

- potty or big toilet
- now or after a song
- step stool or mummy's help
- iPad or music
- "Do you want to flush?" or "Should I?"

These are not small questions.

They are quiet messages that say:

- You matter
- You have a say in your body
- This is happening *with* you, not *to* you

Choice helps regulate the nervous system and reduce fear. It increases cooperation while building trust and predictability.

Small choices create meaningful progress.

Support the nervous system first.
The bladder follows.

A Final Note for Parents

If your child cries, hides, refuses, has accidents, or seems to forget everything — it does not mean the routine isn't working.

It means their nervous system needs time.
Safety is still forming.
Trust is still deepening.
Connection is still doing its quiet work.

Progress in toilet learning is not always visible.

Sometimes it looks like pausing.
Sometimes it looks like retreating.
Sometimes it looks like needing you more.

None of this is failure.

Your bond is the method.
Your presence is the progress.

The routine is simply the scaffold your child leans on while their body learns when it feels safe enough to let go.

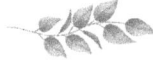

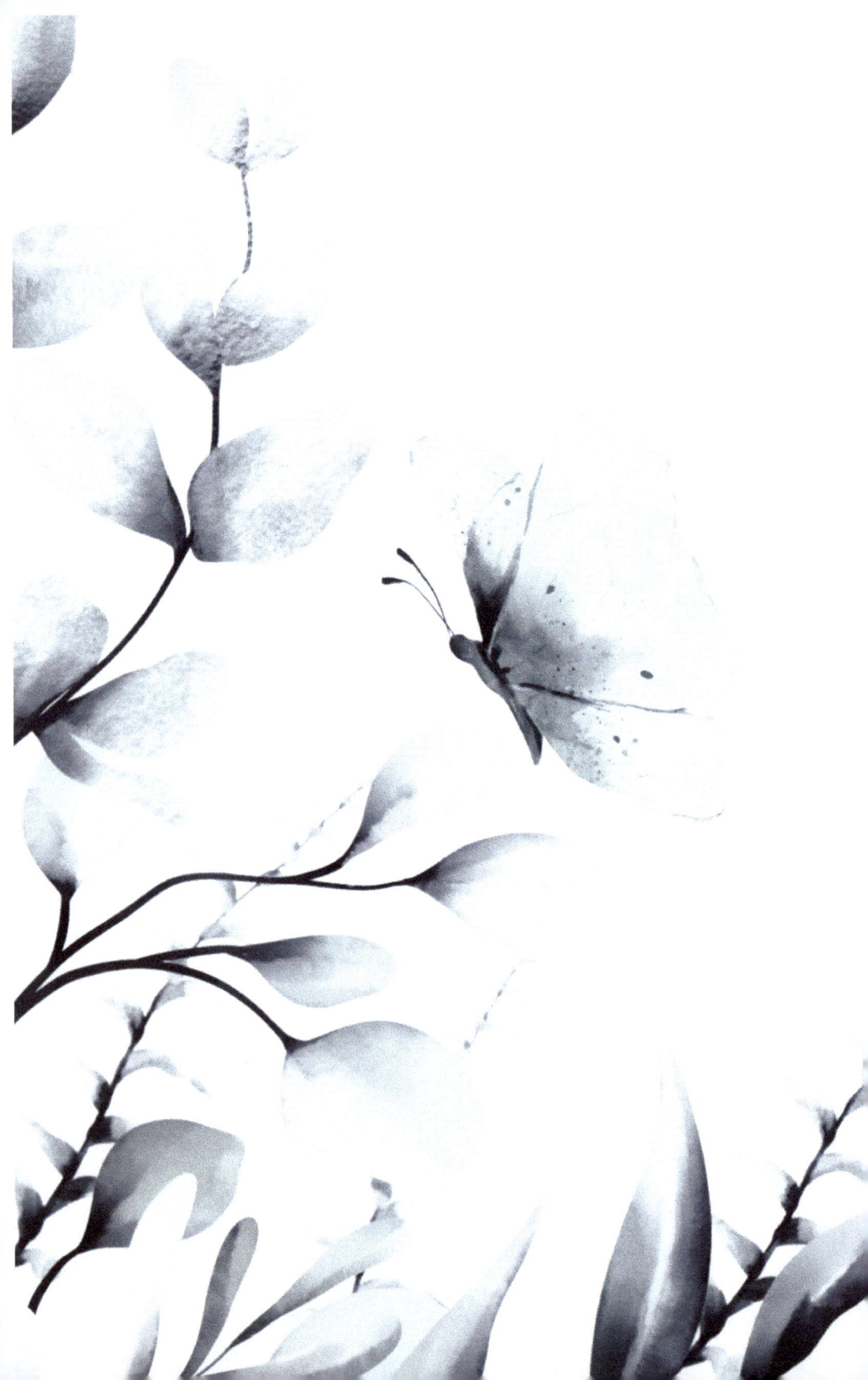

CHAPTER 4

Sitting Without Releasing

One of the most misunderstood parts of toilet learning is sitting on the toilet... and nothing happening.

Many children will happily sit on the toilet long before they ever wee or poo in it. They climb up. They settle in. They chat. They sing. They sit... and nothing happens.

This stage can feel confusing and worrying for parents — especially when you've committed to the process and are quietly waiting for that first release. It can feel like everything is paused. Like you're doing the work, but not seeing the reward.

But sitting without releasing is not a failure.

It is not resistance.

And it is not a sign your child won't learn.

It is a very real and very important stage of toilet learning.

For many children, this is where trust is built. Where safety is established. Where the body begins to learn that this new place is okay.

This stage is foundation, not failure.

Why Sitting Comes Before Releasing

Sitting is something a child can choose.

Releasing is something the body must feel safe enough to do.

Releasing is not a conscious skill. It cannot be taught through instruction or encouragement alone. It relies on the body being ready — on:

• neurological readiness
• relaxed muscles

- emotional safety
- trust in the environment
- clear, recognisable body signals

A child can understand the toilet, want to use it, and still be unable to let go.

For many children, the toilet needs to become familiar before it becomes functional. They need time to sit, observe, and experience the space without expectation.

Learning happens through repetition without pressure. The body must learn the feeling before it can respond to it.

This stage is especially common for children who are sensitive, cautious, neurodivergent, late-talking, deeply body-aware, or highly observant.

These children often learn carefully and thoroughly. Their bodies take longer to soften — not because they are unwilling, but because they are listening closely.

And when the body is ready, releasing often follows with surprising ease.

The Body Needs to Relax Before It Can Release

For wee or poo to come out, the body must relax.

This is not something a child can force. It happens when the body feels safe enough to soften.

Relaxation looks like:

- a soft tummy
- relaxed shoulders
- an unclenched jaw
- a calm, settled nervous system

When a child feels watched, rushed, timed, praised too intensely, or gently pressured to "just try," their body often tightens — even when they are trying their very best.

A tense body cannot release.

Interestingly, the more we want it to happen, the harder it can become.

This is why comfort matters so much at this stage.

Simple supports can help the body soften:

- offering a small toy or book
- letting them watch something familiar
- keeping your voice low and calm
- slowing the moment down
- sitting beside them, not over them

Being close without hovering helps children feel safe.

Comfort is not distraction — it is regulation.

What your child is learning here is not just how to wee or poo. They are learning that the toilet is a safe place for their body.

And safety is what allows release.

Sitting Is Still Learning

When your child sits on the toilet — even without releasing — they are learning.

They are learning where to go.

They are practising the routine.

They are building familiarity.

They are trusting the setup.

They are tuning in to their body.

This is progress.

Sitting itself is a skill.

For some children, sitting can feel regulating one moment and overwhelming the next. It asks their body to pause, to be still, and to notice sensations they are only just beginning to recognise.

Every calm sit teaches something important:

• This place is safe.
• I can pause here.
• My body is okay here.

That learning matters just as much as release.

Short, relaxed sits are far more effective than long, pressured ones.

If your child wants to get down, let them.

Trust grows when your child feels in control of their body and their choices.

Even when nothing comes out, the nervous system is still learning to trust.

Each sit lays another layer of safety.

Sitting without releasing is not wasted time — it is the bridge between awareness and action.

And bridges are built slowly, one steady step at a time.

Charlie's Story

For Charlie, sitting came long before releasing.

She was happy to climb up onto the toilet. She would sit and chat. Sometimes she would talk about wee and poo while she sat there, relaxed and present.

But nothing would come out.

She didn't rush. She didn't resist. And she didn't seem bothered if she was wet later.

From the outside, it could have looked like nothing was happening.

But her body was learning quietly.

Bare-bottom time made it easy for her to sit when a sensation appeared, even if release didn't follow yet.

Sitting became familiar, safe, and pressure-free.

Her awareness came before her motivation.

Charlie showed us that sitting without releasing wasn't a sign of being stuck — it was simply her body learning in the order it needed.

Bare-Bottom Time and Training Pants

For many children in this stage, how connected they feel to their body matters more than anything.

Bare-bottom time can be incredibly supportive because it allows children to feel sensations more clearly — without anything getting in the way.

It can:

- increase awareness of early body signals
- remove barriers between urge and action
- make it easier to sit quickly when a feeling appears
- help children connect what they feel with where it goes

Training pants can also be a helpful bridge.

Unlike nappies, they don't absorb instantly. This allows children to feel wetness and begin to notice what their body is doing — without shame or pressure.

Some children have learned to release only in nappies, simply because nappies feel safe and familiar.

Bare-bottom time or training pants gently interrupt that pattern, while still respecting your child's sense of safety.

Many families naturally move between:

- bare-bottom time at home
- training pants for outings
- nappies for sleep

This flexibility supports learning while protecting emotional safety.

There is no single "right" combination — only what helps your child feel safe enough to learn.

"They Don't Care If They're Wet"

Some children don't react strongly to being wet.

This can worry parents — especially when it feels like caring should come first.

But not caring yet does not mean your child doesn't understand, and it does not mean they won't learn.

For many children — especially those who are sensory-different, deeply absorbed in play, or slower to register body signals — wetness simply isn't uncomfortable enough yet to prompt change.

Awareness comes before motivation.

Caring comes later.

Before children can care about staying dry, they need time to learn:

• what the sensation feels like
• where wee and poo belong
• how to get themselves to the toilet

Some children will tell you with words.

Others will show you through pauses, glances, or small changes in behaviour.

Listening to your child — and noticing which cues are starting to emerge — helps you support them without rushing this stage.

Not caring yet is not a problem.

It is part of the learning process.

And when awareness catches up, caring often follows naturally.

When They Sit, Get Up, Then Wee

Many children will sit on the toilet, climb down... and then wee moments later.

This can be frustrating to witness — especially when it feels like they were so close.

But this is not defiance.

And it is not your child choosing not to use the toilet.

It often happens because:

• the body signal arrived late
• the pressure of sitting made release harder
• standing allowed the body to relax
• movement helped the muscles let go

For many children, especially early in toilet learning, release happens after tension drops.

The important part is not where the wee came out — it's that your child noticed the sensation and allowed it to happen.

If you can, simply guide them back to the toilet and say:

"Let's finish wee wee on the toilet."

This gently connects the feeling with the place.

You can offer a calm, neutral encouragement:

"Good job."

Then move on.

No shame.
No disappointment.
No urgency.

Just information and connection.

This moment is still learning.

Each time it happens, your child's body is mapping the sequence:

feeling → movement → release → meaning

And with time, those steps begin to line up.

The Fear: "What If They Never Get It?"

This is often the hardest part of this stage.

Your child is trying. You're doing everything "right." And still, nothing seems to change.

Progress feels invisible.

A quiet fear creeps in:

What if they never get it?

This fear is incredibly common.

And it makes sense.

When learning is happening on the inside, it can feel like you're standing still — waiting, watching, wondering if you should be doing more or something differently.

But toilet learning rarely looks like steady progress.

It often looks like a long pause, followed by sudden change.

At this stage, your child isn't deciding whether to learn — their body is still organising the signals it needs to feel safe enough to release.

That work is quiet.

It doesn't show up as success right away.

You are asked to trust what you cannot yet see.

To stay calm while nothing appears to be moving.

To keep showing up with steadiness instead of urgency.

Children do not miss this milestone forever.

When the body is ready, release often comes suddenly — sometimes after weeks that felt unchanged.

This stage feels long because the learning is happening underneath the surface.

You are not stuck.

Your child is not behind.

You are standing in the middle — where trust is built, even when confidence wobbles.

The 2–12 Week Window

Toilet learning is not a three-day process for most children.

For many families, it unfolds gently over 2–12 weeks.

This timeframe is not a rule or a deadline — it is a guiding window that reflects how long bodies often need to learn something new.

This time allows space for:

• clearer body signals to emerge
• muscles to relax and coordinate
• routines to feel familiar
• confidence to build
• trust to grow

Children who sit without releasing are often in the early-to-middle part of this window.

This does not mean they are behind.

It means their body is still integrating what it has learned.

For many children, everything comes together quietly — and then suddenly.

Progress doesn't always announce itself.

Sometimes it shows up all at once.

Signs Release May Be Coming Soon

Progress in this stage is often quiet and easy to miss.

Many parents assume release will come with clear signals — but for most children, it arrives after a series of small, subtle shifts.

Signs your child may be getting closer include:

• sitting for longer without prompting
• talking about wee or poo more often
• naming or noticing sensations
• pausing briefly during play
• holding themselves for a moment
• sitting, getting up, then releasing
• choosing the toilet independently
• copying the language you use around toileting

These are not random behaviours.

They are signs the body is carefully mapping the process.

For many children, release comes suddenly — after weeks that looked unchanged from the outside.

What feels like "nothing happening" is often the final stretch of integration.

A Gentle Reminder Before Moving On

If your child is:

- sitting willingly
- calm on the toilet
- engaged with the process
- showing no signs of distress

Then you are not stuck.

You are in the quiet middle — the place where learning deepens before it becomes visible.

This stage does not end because you push harder.

It ends because your child's body finally feels safe enough to let go.

And safety is something you are already giving.

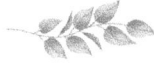

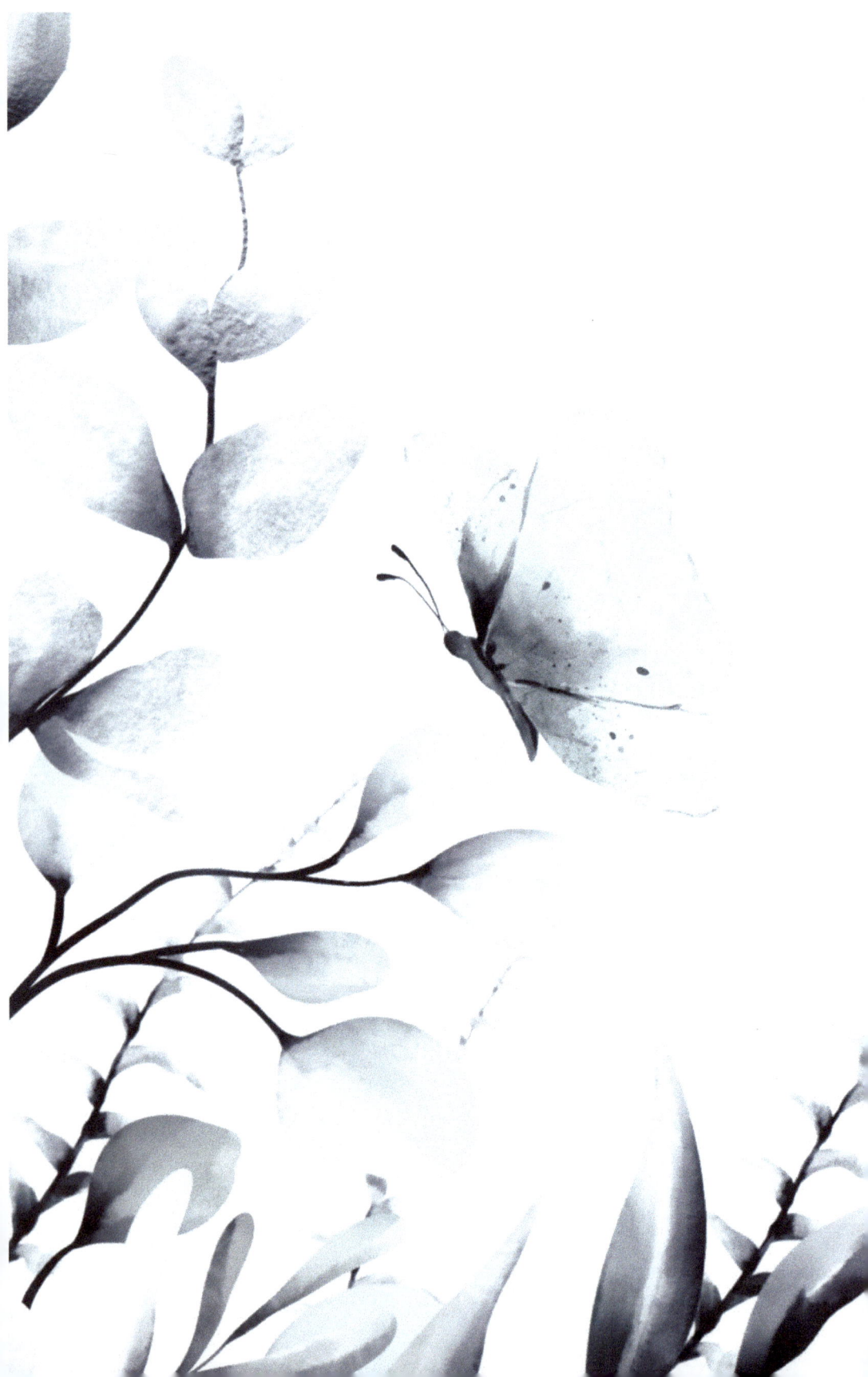

CHAPTER 5

The Middle Journey & the Quiet Wins

There is a part of toilet learning that almost no one talks about.

It's the middle.

Not the beginning — where everything feels intentional and hopeful.
Not the end — where skills feel settled and confidence has arrived.

But the long, quiet stretch in between.

This is the part where progress is happening... but it doesn't always look like progress.
Where days blur together.
Where your child seems capable one moment and uninterested the next.

Where you start wondering if you're doing something wrong — or if you've somehow stalled the process.

This is the middle journey.
And it is where most toilet learning actually happens.

The Middle Is Not a Plateau

The middle can feel like nothing is changing.

Your child might:

• sit confidently but still not release
• use the toilet once... then not again for days
• tell you when they've weed after it's happened
• seem less enthusiastic than they were at the start
• have accidents after what felt like a breakthrough

This can feel discouraging — especially if you were expecting steady forward movement.

But the middle is not a plateau.

It is an integration phase.

Your child's body and brain are quietly:

- mapping sensations
- practising control
- learning timing
- building trust
- strengthening independence
- deciding when they feel ready

These changes happen beneath the surface.
And they take time.

When the 'Keen' Phase Fades

For many children, the early "keen" phase is actually the novelty phase.

Those children you hear about who "do it in three days" are often riding a mix of:

- novelty
- adult focus
- subtle pressure
- adrenaline

That early excitement is common — and it fades for almost all children, even the fast ones.

You just don't usually hear about the flat days that follow.

When novelty wears off, learning shifts from something external to something internal.

And internal learning looks quieter.
Slower.
Less performative.

So when a child seems "not as keen," it doesn't mean they've stopped learning.

It usually means their brain has moved from showing to integrating.

Some Children Learn Thoughtfully, Not Loudly

Not all children charge through learning.

Some children:

• notice first
• think carefully

- notice first
- think carefully
- check safety
- feel their way through
- and only then act

These children often:

- initiate less when tired
- pause when overwhelmed
- resist when expectations feel heavy
- step back when something feels emotionally loaded

This isn't delay.
And it isn't refusal.

It's a sensitive, regulated nervous system doing exactly what it's meant to do.

Children like this still learn — they just do it in a way that is quieter, more deliberate, and deeply rooted in safety.

A Real-Life Moment from the Middle

At this stage, one child would happily climb onto the toilet, settle in, chat away, and talk confidently about wee and poo — yet still not release.

She wasn't avoiding the toilet.
She wasn't afraid.
She wasn't resisting.

She was thinking.

Some days she initiated on her own.
Other days she stepped back.

She showed awareness, comfort, and understanding long before her body was ready to let go.

What helped most wasn't more encouragement or longer sits — it was allowing her to move at her own pace, without turning the toilet into a performance.

In time, her body caught up to what her mind already knew.

This is what thoughtful learning can look like.

The Quiet Wins Matter

Quiet wins are easy to miss — especially when you're tired, watching closely, and hoping for reassurance.

But they matter just as much as the first wee in the toilet.

Quiet wins include:

• sitting willingly, even briefly
• choosing the toilet independently
• staying dry for longer stretches
• talking about wee or poo
• letting you know after an accident
• helping with undressing
• wanting privacy
• returning to the toilet after getting up
• saying "next time" or "try again"

These moments tell you something important:

Your child is learning.

Even if nothing made it into the toilet today.

Why Comparison Can Make This Harder

It's hard not to compare.

But it's important to know this:

The "three-day" children are not the standard.

They sit outside the usual pattern.

Most Children:

• take weeks
• have dips after progress
• lose enthusiasm
• regain it later
• plateau
• need pauses

And children who have:

• delayed or subtle body signals
• speech or processing differences
• high emotional attunement

almost never follow a fast or linear timeline — and that is not a problem.

Comparison doesn't speed learning.
It usually just increases pressure.

And pressure is what sensitive children feel most.

A Reframe for the Spiral Moments

When the worry loop starts, it often sounds like this:

Why hasn't my child weed in the toilet yet?

A more helpful question is:

What skills does my child have now that they didn't have before?

Awareness.
Initiation.
Comfort.
Understanding.
Safety.

When you list them, the progress becomes clearer.

You're not trying to convince yourself of something untrue.
 You're reminding yourself of what's actually happening.

When Pulling Back Is the Most Supportive Move

When toilet learning becomes:

• talked about constantly

• watched closely

• emotionally charged

some children instinctively step back.

Not because they don't want to learn — but because they need control and safety again.

This can show up as:

• less eagerness

• more holding

• quieter engagement

• resistance to sitting

This isn't a sign to push harder.

It's a signal to soften.

Often the most supportive shift at this stage is:

- fewer reminders
- more neutral language
- less sitting "for the sake of it"
- more following your child's lead
- more "it's there if you want it"

You're not stopping the process.
You're lowering the emotional load so readiness can return naturally.

Trusting a Slow Process

Children who take longer at the start often have fewer issues later.

They aren't pushed past their nervous system.
They learn once — properly — and then move on.

Supporting a child this way is not easy.

It means:

- trusting a slow process
- resisting pressure

- staying emotionally available
- leading without forcing

That takes strength.

You don't need to rush your child's body.
You don't need to fix the timeline.

You just need to keep doing what you're already doing — steady, kind, observant, patient.

A Gentle Reminder for Parents

If you're in the middle of this journey and it feels heavy, pause for a moment.

Two weeks is nothing in body-learning time.
Quiet progress is still progress.
Delayed signals don't mean "won't learn" — they mean "learns differently."

When your thoughts spiral, try asking:

What can my child do now that they couldn't do before?

The answer is usually more than you realise.

You don't need to rush their body.

You don't need to fix the timeline.

You just need to keep offering what you already are:

Safety.

Steadiness.

Patience.

Trust.

And on the days it feels hard, you're allowed to say that out loud.

This process doesn't ask you to be perfect — it asks you to be present.

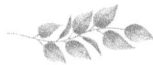

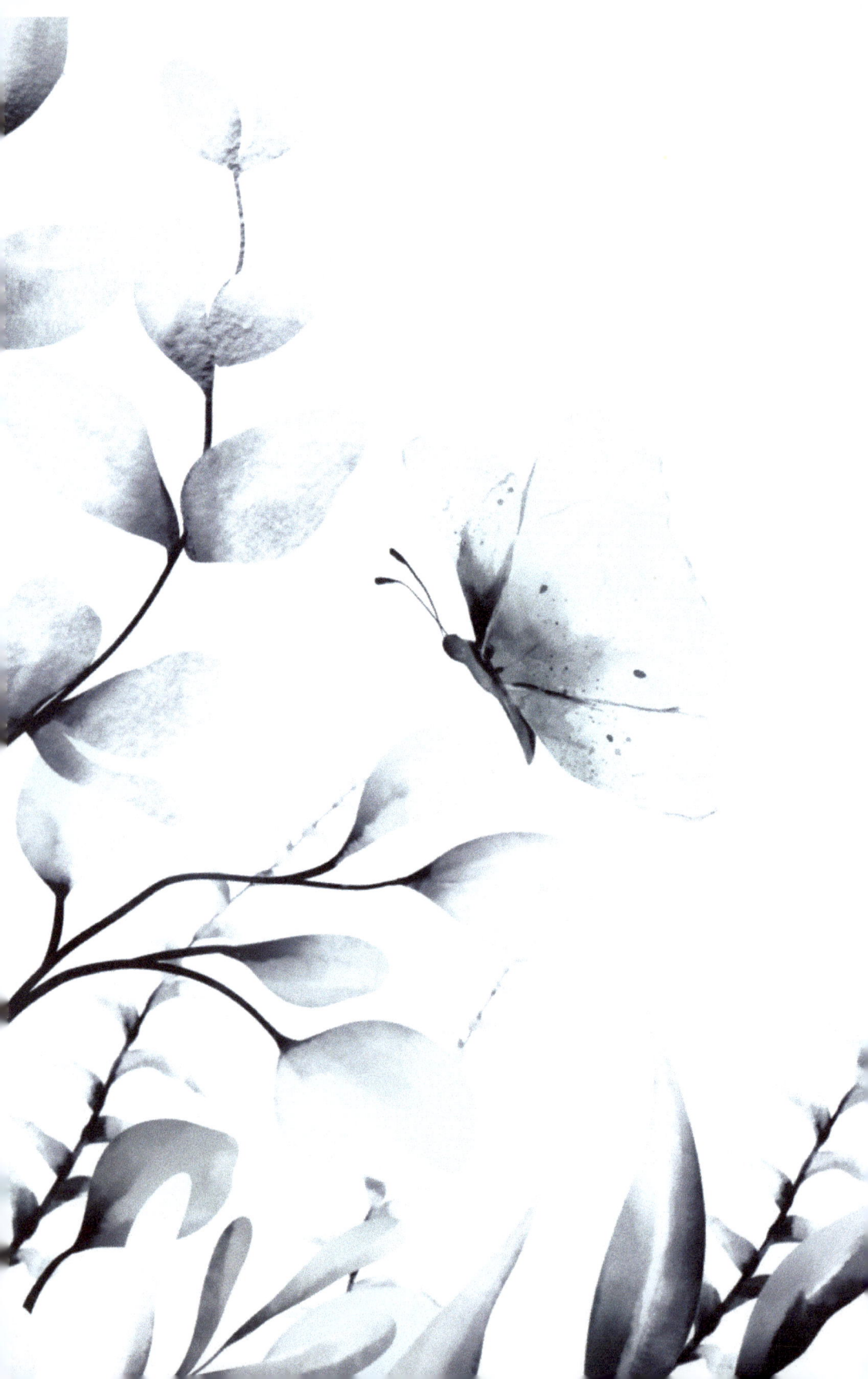

CHAPTER 6

The Power of Words and Connection

The words you use during toilet learning become part of how your child feels about their body. Your language shapes whether this experience feels safe or stressful, calm or pressured, supportive or overwhelming.

Often without realising it, the way we speak — our tone, our timing, even our pauses — tells our child what this learning space is like. Is it a place where they can relax? Or a place where their body feels watched, rushed, or unsure?

Toilet learning is not just about what a child does with their body. It's about how their body feels while they're learning. It lives in your tone. In your presence. In the sense of safety you bring into the moment.

For many children — especially sensitive, observant, or neurodivergent children, and children who don't thrive under pressure — learning doesn't begin with action. It begins with connection. With feeling close. With feeling understood. With knowing they are safe with you — exactly as they are — even before anything "happens."

Connection is what settles a child's nervous system. It allows the body to soften instead of brace. When a child feels safe, their body isn't busy protecting itself. It isn't holding, guarding, or waiting for the moment to pass. Instead, the body can slow down. Notice sensations. Learn what it needs to learn in its own time.

This is why connection matters so much in toilet learning. Because when that sense of safety is there, the body has space to learn — and learning can unfold gently, without force.

<u>Words Shape the Body's Response</u>

Children don't separate skills from feelings. They experience learning through relationship. They're not just listening to what we say — they're sensing how it feels to be with us in that moment.

So the language used around toileting doesn't just land in their ears. It lands in their body.

When a child feels watched, rushed, or expected to perform, their body often responds by tightening. Muscles hold. Breathing becomes shallow. The body shifts into protection mode.

Pressure tightens the body.
Expectation creates holding.
Urgency interrupts release.

Even when it's subtle. Even when it's well-intentioned. Even when we're trying to help.

Safety does the opposite.

When a child feels emotionally safe — when they feel accepted, unhurried, and supported — their body can soften. Breathing slows. Sensations become easier to notice. This is when learning becomes possible. Not because the child is trying harder — but because their body no longer needs to protect itself.

If you've noticed your child holding more when things feel tense, this isn't a setback — it's communication.

In a safe emotional space, the body can relax, tune in, and eventually let go in its own time.

This is why words matter so much. Not because the "right words" teach the skill — but because your tone, your presence, and your response shape the environment in which the skill is allowed to emerge.

Connection Before Correction

Before a child can coordinate muscles, timing, and sensation, their nervous system needs to feel settled. That sense of calm doesn't come from explanation or instruction. It comes from presence.

Connection helps a child's body feel safe enough to stay in the moment. It tells them they're not being watched, tested, or evaluated. It tells them they don't have to get it "right."

When we move too quickly into correcting or prompting — even with the best intentions — a child's body can tighten. Learning becomes something to perform rather than something to explore.

Connection shifts that completely.

Connection looks like:

• sitting nearby without expectation
• chatting without an agenda
• letting the moment be what it is
• staying warm and steady, even when nothing "happens"

It might look like sitting together on the bathroom floor. Or sharing a quiet conversation while they sit. Or simply being there — calm, unhurried, and emotionally available.

In these moments, you're not missing a teaching opportunity. You're creating the conditions that make learning possible.

Connection tells the body:

"I'm safe here."

"I'm not being rushed."

"I don't have to perform."

If you've ever worried that you're not doing enough because you're not correcting or prompting, this is your reassurance: your calm presence is doing the work.

Safety is what allows learning to continue. And connection is how safety is built.

What Learning Can Look Like (Even When Nothing Is "Happening")

Sometimes, progress doesn't look like release. Sometimes, nothing obvious happens at all — and yet learning is unfolding right in front of you.

It can look like this:

- She comes into the toilet space with you.
- She's comfortable enough to chat.
- She uses the words "poo" and "wee."
- She connects the idea: toilet = poo/wee.
- There's ease in her body.
- No tension. No urgency.
- She's not avoiding.
- She's not disengaged.
- She's not failing to try.

She's understanding.

That quiet moment — easy to overlook — tells us something important.

This is cognitive understanding paired with emotional safety.

For some children, learning happens like this:

Do the wee → Then understand it

But for many children — especially those who are sensitive, observant, body-aware, or who don't thrive under pressure — learning unfolds differently:

Understand it

Feel safe with it

Talk about it

Sit near it

Sit on it

Then, when the body is ready, release

This is not a delay. It's a different pathway.

A pathway that honours how deeply these children need to feel safe before their body can act.

When a child talks about wee and poo while you're on the toilet, they're often saying:

"I know what this place is for."

"I understand what happens here."

"I'm just not ready to do my part yet."

And that's okay.

Understanding often comes before release.

If this feels like your child, you're not behind. This stage isn't wasted time. It's the groundwork.

And release will come — when the body feels safe enough to follow the mind.

Language That Supports Learning

Supportive language focuses on process, not outcomes. It lets your child know their effort matters — even when their body hasn't done what they hoped yet.

Supportive language might sound like:

- "You're listening to your body."
- "You noticed that feeling."
- "Thank you for sitting."
- "Thank you for trying."
- "You gave it a go."

These words tell your child:

Trying is enough.

You're not doing this wrong.

You can also offer simple, neutral information:

- "Wee wee goes in the toilet."
- "It's okay to relax and wee."

- "You're safe to wee here."
- "Your body lets wee out when it's ready."

When nothing happens:

- "It's okay."
- "We can try again another time."
- "Your body is still learning."

And gently, without pressure:

- "Next time we'll try to wee in the toilet."
- "Next time your body might tell you earlier."

For children who release after leaving the toilet, this language matters deeply. It tells them:

You're still learning.
You're still on the right path.
Nothing went wrong.

They don't need more reminders. They need more safety.

When Accidents Happen

Accidents are not mistakes. They are information.

They're your child's body saying, "I'm still learning."

When accidents happen, a child's nervous system is already vulnerable. They may feel surprised or unsure. They look to you to understand what it means.

This is where calm matters most.

A calm response might sound like:

- "You did wee."
- "Your wee came out then."
- "Your body let go."

From there, gentle redirection can happen:

- "Let's finish the wee on the toilet."
- "Wee goes in the toilet."
- "Let's take the rest to the toilet together."

Once things are settled, you might gently reflect:

- "Did you feel that pressure before the wee came out?"
- "Sometimes our body tells us a bit late."
- "Next time your body might tell you earlier."

These aren't tests. They're invitations to notice.

And sometimes, cleaning up quietly together is enough.

After an accident, what your child needs most is safety:

- "It's okay."
- "Your body is learning."
- "Nothing went wrong."

A child who feels safe after an accident stays open to learning.

Connection Beyond the Toilet

Connection doesn't only live in the bathroom.

Much of the learning that supports toileting happens in quiet, everyday moments — in shared closeness, gentle routines, and the way your child feels with you throughout the day.

Connection fills your child's emotional cup. It helps their nervous system settle. It tells their body that it's safe enough to learn.

For many children, emotional safety is built long before they ever sit on the toilet.

It's built in morning snuggles before the day begins.
In sitting close on the couch.
In being nearby while you cook dinner.
In your child following you from room to room — not because they need something, but because they need you.

These moments might feel ordinary. Easy to overlook. Easy to rush.

But they matter.

They're how your child regulates.
How they steady themselves.
How their body prepares for new challenges.

Children who seek closeness aren't being needy. They're regulating.

And when that need is met, confidence grows quietly. Their body doesn't have to cling so tightly. Their independence comes when it's ready.

Connection is not a detour from independence.

It's the road that leads to it.

You Are the Safe Place

Your child isn't learning toileting on their own.

They're learning it *with you.*

In the way you stay close.
In the way you speak softly.
In the way you don't rush the moment, even when you're tired or unsure.

Every time you choose calm over pressure, connection over correction, you are offering your child something far bigger than a skill.

You are offering safety.

If toilet learning feels slow, it doesn't mean you're behind.
If progress feels quiet or uneven, it doesn't mean nothing is happening.

If your child needs more time, more closeness, more reassurance — that isn't a problem to fix.

It's a need being met.

You don't need perfect words.
You don't need to get every moment right.

Your presence is already enough.

Learning will come — not because you forced it, but because you made it safe to arrive.

And that safety is something your child will carry with them long after this season has passed.

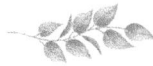

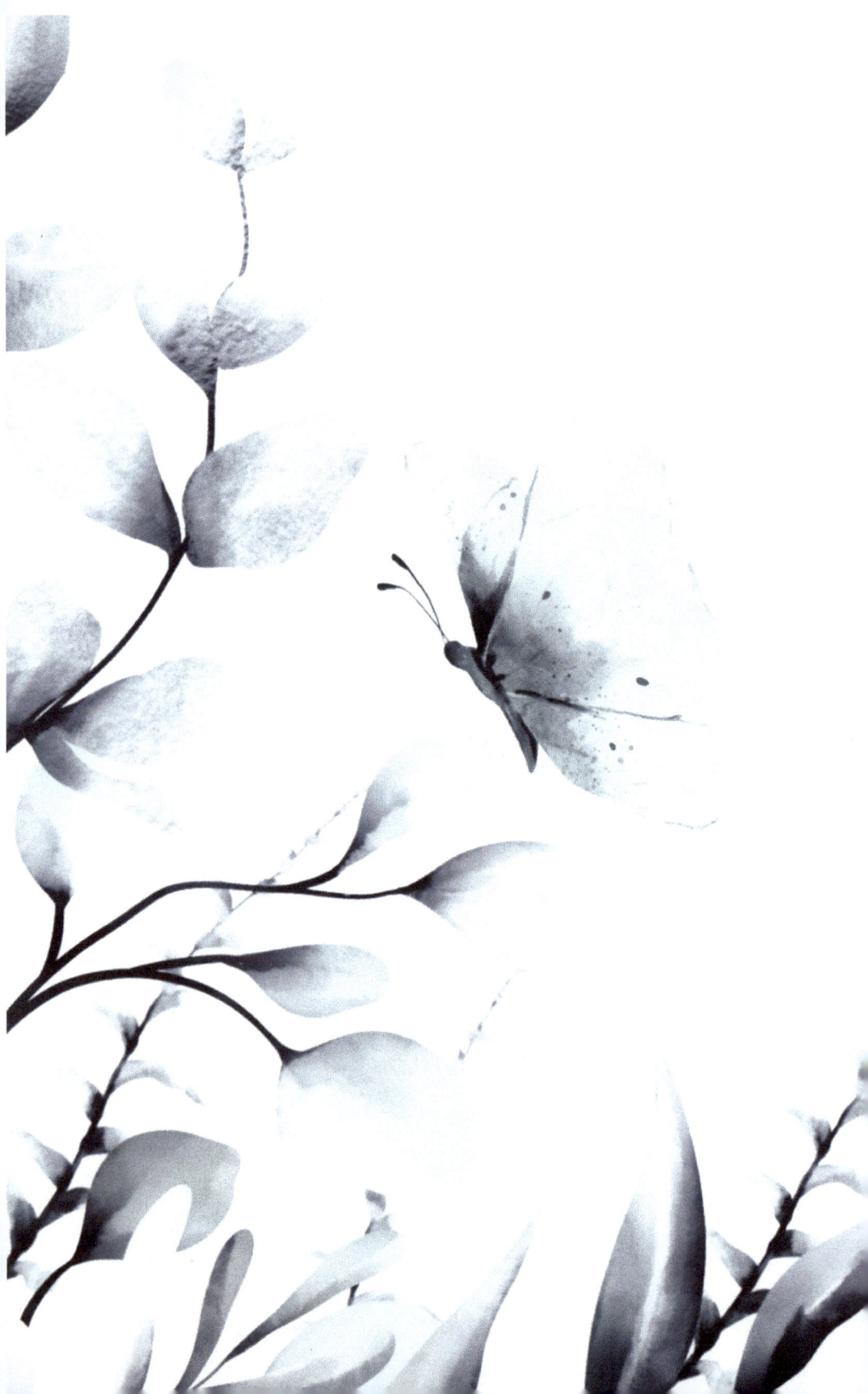

Chapter 7

Troubleshooting Difficult Moments

A Gentle Guide When Things Feel Stuck

B efore we troubleshoot anything, parents need to hear this:

If toilet learning feels hard right now, you haven't failed. You're simply listening to a child whose body is still learning. It's okay if you're having hard moments too. It's okay to feel unsure, emotional, or tired of thinking about the toilet.

This chapter isn't here to add pressure. It's here to help you understand what might be getting in the way — so you can move forward with more ease, trust, and steadiness.

Foundation First (Read This Before Fixing Anything)

When toileting feels stuck, it can help to gently pause before trying to change anything.

Toilet learning doesn't happen in isolation. It's shaped by how safe a child feels, how regulated their body is, and what their nervous system can manage on any given day. These things can shift — even when nothing obvious has.

If progress feels slow or unclear, it doesn't mean something is wrong. Often, it means something needs a little more care.

These questions can help you slow down and listen:

Is my child feeling emotionally safe right now?
Emotional safety comes from feeling accepted, unhurried, and not evaluated. When a child feels safe, their body is more able to let go.

Does their body seem relaxed enough to release?
A tense or busy body will often hold on — even when a

child wants to wee. Relaxation can't be forced; it grows from comfort and familiarity.

Am I expecting more than their nervous system can manage today?
Illness, tiredness, change, sensory overload, or big emotions can all reduce what a child has available for learning.

If any of these feel like a "not quite," progress may slow or pause for a while — and that's okay.

Pauses don't mean learning has stopped. They often mean the body is gathering itself before moving forward again.

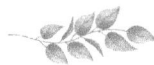

1. My Child Sits on the Toilet but Nothing Happens

This is one of the most common — and confusing — moments in toilet learning.

Your child may already be developing body awareness, but learning when and how to release in a new position takes time. Sitting on a toilet asks the body to coordinate muscles in a new way, and for many children this develops gradually. Sometimes the nervous system is still deciding whether this place feels safe enough to let go.

What can help:

• Softening expectations ("You don't have to wee — you're just sitting")
• Keeping sits short and relaxed
• Offering privacy or stepping away
• Remembering that learning doesn't only happen on the toilet — floor wees and familiar places can be part of the bridge

Nothing is wasted here. The body is still learning.

2. My Child Understands Everything but Still Wees Elsewhere

This can feel especially hard, because it looks like your child knows what to do.

But understanding comes before body readiness. A child can know the routine, the language, and the goal while their body is still learning how to act on early signals.

For many children, release is still reflex-based. Signals may arrive too late to move in time — and that's developmental, not defiance.

What can help:

- Bare-bottom time to make sensations clearer
- Calm, neutral clean-ups
- Treating accidents as information, not problems
- Time — often more time than we expect

Learning is still happening, even when it's messy.

3. Pulling Pants or Undies Down Seems to Stop the Wee

This is very common, even though it's rarely talked about.

Pulling pants or undies down is a skill in itself. Even when a child already knows how to do it, connecting that skill to noticing a body signal, moving to the toilet, balancing, sitting, and then releasing is a lot for a little person to coordinate.

Sometimes the body knows it needs to wee, but as soon as the focus shifts to doing the steps, the moment is interrupted. The attention moves from "my body needs to wee" to "I need to do this properly." When that happens, the body can tighten — and the wee disappears.

This doesn't mean your child isn't capable. It often means their brain and body are still learning how to link these skills together.

What can help:

• Practising pulling pants down outside toilet moments
• Choosing looser, easy-to-manage clothing
• Returning to bare-bottom time if that feels

supportive

• Treating pants as something that comes later, not all at once

Simplifying isn't going backwards. It's often what clears the path forward.

4. My Child Was Progressing, Then Stopped — or Refuses to Sit

This can be one of the most worrying moments for parents.

Things may have been moving along — small signs, curiosity, willingness — and then your child pauses, resists, or starts saying "no." It can feel confusing, discouraging, and emotionally heavy.

Often, what looks like stopping is actually integration. Developmental leaps, illness, tiredness, big emotions, changes in routine, or increased expectations can all slow progress for a while. Sometimes a child's nervous system is simply busy processing something else.

For some children, that pause shows up as refusal. Refusal can feel confronting, but it's often communication. Saying "no" can be a way of protecting autonomy while things reorganise internally.

What can help:

• Reconnecting through play, closeness, and everyday moments
• Reducing toilet talk for a few days
• Offering choices instead of instructions
• Letting the toilet exist without focus

Learning doesn't disappear. It often settles quietly before finding its way back.

Refusal isn't defiance. It's information.

5. My Child Only Wees at School or Childcare (or Only at Home)

It can be surprising — and sometimes worrying — when your child wees confidently in one place but not in another.

Different environments create different feelings of safety. Routines, expectations, sounds, people, and even how the toilet is used can all affect how relaxed a child's body feels.

This split is very common, especially for sensitive or observant children.

What can help:

• Letting go of comparisons
• Gently aligning language across settings where possible
• Allowing each environment to support learning in its own way

Consistency matters — and emotional safety matters just as much.

If you find yourself worrying that school or childcare is "doing it better," please remember — your child isn't choosing sides. They're responding to how safe their body feels in that moment, and your relationship is still their anchor.

6. Frequent Accidents — or Understanding Without Making It in Time

Frequent accidents, or weeing away from the toilet even though your child seems to understand what to do, can feel discouraging and exhausting.

It can look like "they know what to do, but just aren't doing it." More often, it simply means learning is still unfolding at a body level.

When accidents are happening often

Frequent accidents are usually a sign that learning is underway — not that it's failing. Body signals may still be forming, or release may happen very quickly once it begins. For some children, there's only a small gap between noticing the sensation and needing to release.

Body awareness grows through experience, not through getting it right every time.

When your child understands but still wees elsewhere

Understanding often comes before body readiness. A child can know the routine, the words, and the goal while their body is still learning how to act on early signals.

For many children, release is still reflex-based. Signals may arrive too late to move in time — and that's developmental, not defiance.

Both of these experiences sit in the same learning window: the body is still working out when and how to respond.

What can help:

- Calm, neutral responses and clean-ups
- Fewer reminders and less prompting
- Observing rather than asking
- Bare-bottom time to make sensations clearer
- Letting accidents gently teach timing
- Treating accidents as information, not problems
- Time — often more time than we expect

Learning is still happening, even when it's messy.

Frequent accidents don't mean you missed a window. They mean the body is still learning.

7. My Child Seems Anxious, Upset, or Holds On Around the Toilet

When a child seems anxious, upset, or holds on around the toilet, it's something worth pausing with.

Distress — including holding on — is often your child's way of telling you they need more safety. It's rarely about refusal or stubbornness. More often, the body is doing its best to protect itself.

Some children feel unsure when they're being watched or waited on, even when encouragement is gentle. Others are still working out what release feels like in this new position, or may find the sensations unfamiliar or uncomfortable.

When this happens, it doesn't mean your child isn't ready to learn. It usually means they need more time, space, or reassurance.

What can help:

- Giving space or privacy
- Using neutral, low-key language
- Gently shifting attention
- Letting the sit be just sitting, with no expectation

If distress is showing up, easing off toilet focus and rebuilding connection through everyday moments can help restore safety.

Reassuring your child that they're not in trouble, and that their body is okay, can be deeply settling.

If anxiety or distress continues over time, reaching out for extra support can be a gentle next step.

Emotional safety always comes first.

If you're carrying worry that you caused this, be gentle with yourself. That worry is a sign of care, not a mistake.

8. Low-Pressure Days (A Reset, Not a Step Back)

Low-pressure days aren't giving up. They're a way of listening.

Sometimes, when toileting starts to feel tense, the most supportive thing you can do is stop trying to move things forward for a moment.

Low-pressure days give your child's nervous system a break from being noticed, measured, or waited on. For many children, especially sensitive or highly observant ones, even gentle prompting can begin to feel like expectation. When that happens, the body often responds by holding on.

A low-pressure day might mean:

• Less prompting
• Fewer reminders
• Less checking in
• Very little or no toilet talk

You still respond if your child initiates — but you don't lead the day with toileting.

For some families, low-pressure days also include using training pants or pull-ups. This can help keep wees off the floor and take practical stress off the parent, without undoing learning.

Low-pressure days aren't just for children. They support parents too.

When pressure eases, both nervous systems get a chance to reset.

These days send a powerful message: "We're okay. There's no rush."

Often, after one or two low-pressure days, things feel lighter. Learning doesn't disappear — it often becomes more accessible because everyone feels calmer.

Low-pressure days aren't about doing nothing. They're about doing less — on purpose.

If today feels heavy — today can be a low-pressure day.

9. It's Been Weeks and We Still Feel Stuck

This is often the hardest point.

The early days are full of hope and energy. The middle can feel uncertain. And then there's this moment — when time has passed, effort has been given, and things still don't feel clear.

This is where many parents begin to doubt themselves.

You might start questioning:

• Am I missing something?
• Did I start too early?
• Am I doing this wrong?
• Why does this seem easier for other families?

If you're here, you're not alone — and you haven't failed.

A Gentle Reminder — and an Important One

Toilet learning commonly takes 2–12 weeks. Sometimes longer.

That time includes learning body sensations, muscle coordination, emotional safety, and trust.

Taking longer doesn't mean something is wrong.

Learning doesn't always look like progress.

Sometimes it looks like waiting.

Sometimes it looks like circling.

Sometimes it looks like nothing at all.

But underneath, your child's body is still gathering information.

If you're still here, still caring — you are not behind. You are inside the process.

Sometimes, this is the moment when more understanding or support can help.

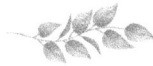

When to Seek Extra Support (And Why It's Okay)

You were never meant to do this alone.

Toilet learning can bring up more emotion, worry, and self-doubt than many parents expect — especially when progress feels slow or unclear.

Reaching out for support doesn't mean you've failed. It means you're paying attention.

It's okay to seek extra help if:

• Stress feels high for you or your child
• Toileting is causing ongoing distress or anxiety
• Progress feels stalled for a long time
• You've tried adjusting your approach and still feel unsure
• Something in your body is telling you there may be more going on

Sometimes, extra support simply helps you see your child more clearly. Other times, it can gently uncover things that aren't obvious on the surface — such as differences in body awareness, sensory processing, communication, muscle coordination, or nervous system regulation.

None of these are anyone's fault.

And none of them mean your child won't learn.

Support doesn't take over your role as a parent. It doesn't replace your instincts. It works alongside you — helping you understand why things might be feeling stuck, and what kind of support your child needs right now.

For some families, a small adjustment makes everything click. For others, having someone walk beside them for a while brings relief and confidence back into the process.

Asking for help isn't giving up. It isn't rushing. And it isn't a sign that you or your child have done something wrong.

It's thoughtful, responsive parenting — and sometimes, it's the most loving step you can take.

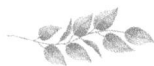

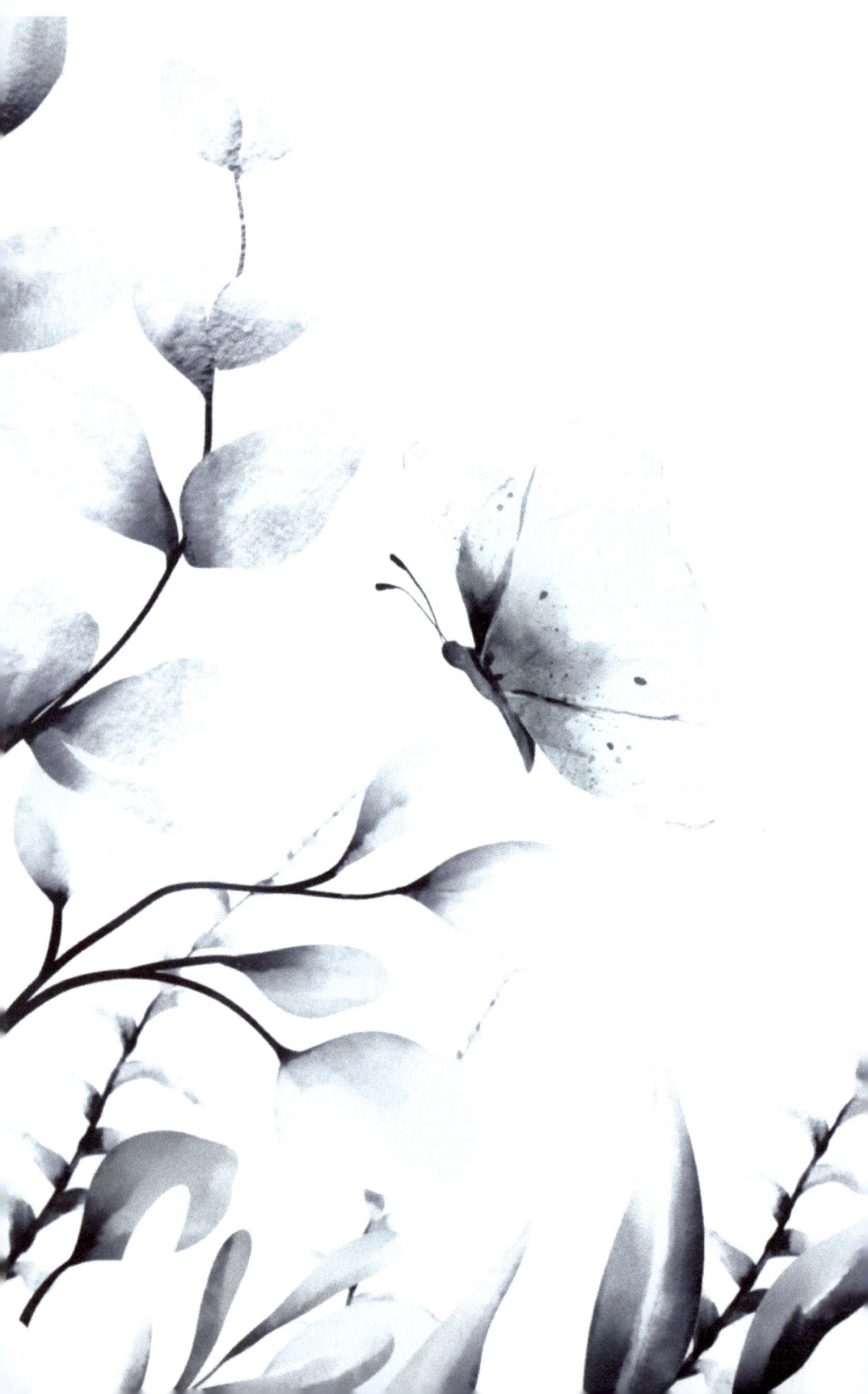

CHAPTER 8

Celebrating Their Kind of Progress

T oilet training is often talked about as a finish line. Dry days. No accidents. Pants on. Done.

But when you're walking this path with a sensitive, late-talking, or neurodivergent child — or a child who simply doesn't thrive under pressure — progress doesn't look like a straight line. And it definitely doesn't look like what most people talk about.

This chapter is about slowing down enough to really see the progress that actually matters. The quiet progress. The invisible progress. The progress that lives inside your child's body, nervous system, confidence, and sense of safety.

It's about noticing the moments that make your heart lift a little. The tiny wins that spark hope. The growth that might not look dramatic — but feels huge when you're the one living it.

Because when you start noticing *their* kind of progress, everything changes.

Progress Is More Than Wee and Poo

Many parents are taught to measure success by just one thing:

Did they wee or poo in the toilet?

And when that doesn't happen, it can quietly chip away at your confidence. It can make you wonder if you're doing something wrong — or if your child is falling behind.

But for many children — especially those who are sensitive, develop differently, or don't respond well to pressure — the real work happens long before anything lands in the bowl.

Sometimes progress looks like your child simply sitting.

Fully clothed.

For a few seconds.

With a body that's still learning to trust.

It might look like:

- Standing in the bathroom doorway, watching you
- Talking about wee or poo without fear
- Letting you know *after* they've done a wee
- Or being willing to try again tomorrow

These moments are not small.

They are not delays.

They are not failures.

They are the building blocks.

Before a child can use the toilet confidently, their body needs to feel safe. Safe enough to pause. Safe enough to sit. Safe enough to stay.

So progress often shows up in the body first — not as results, but as signals:

- Relaxed shoulders instead of tension
- A deep breath
- Staying seated a little longer than last time
- Not rushing to jump off
- Laughing, chatting, or simply *being* on the toilet

If you've ever felt that quiet surge of joy — *They sat!* — you're not imagining it. That moment matters.

Your child's nervous system is learning that the toilet is a safe place. And when safety comes first, everything else follows.

Parent Affirmation

"Sitting, staying, and feeling safe are real wins."

Progress Is Willingness

Willingness is one of the most overlooked — and most powerful — milestones in toilet learning.

Because willingness means your child feels safe enough to engage. It means they're not shutting down. Not bracing. Not protecting themselves from pressure.

Sometimes progress looks like your child walking toward the toilet when you gently suggest it — and that moment alone is worth celebrating.

Willingness might look like:

• Walking to the toilet with you
• Saying "no" calmly instead of melting down
• Agreeing to sit after an accident
• Letting you help with wiping or flushing
• Staying open instead of shutting down
• Trying again after a miss

These moments carry quiet bravery.

They tell you your child is trusting the process — and trusting *you*.

A willing child is a learning child.

And willingness grows when pressure shrinks.

Parent Affirmation

"My child's willingness tells me they feel safe — and safety is where learning begins."

What You Can Say to Your Child
"I'm proud of how you tried."

Progress Is Emotional Safety

Sometimes the biggest progress has nothing to do with the toilet at all.

It looks like:

• Running to you after an accident instead of hiding
• Letting you comfort them
• Laughing it off instead of crying
• Saying "It's okay" after a miss
• Trusting that you won't be upset

These moments tell you something important.

Your child feels safe with you.
Safe enough to be honest.
Safe enough to be imperfect.
Safe enough to keep learning.

That safety reaches far beyond toilet training. It shapes how your child copes, trusts, and believes in themselves.

And that kind of progress is quietly profound.

A Charlie Moment: The Progress I Didn't Expect

There was a day I realised how much progress Charlie had actually made — and it wasn't because she did a wee in the toilet.

She wandered into the bathroom on her own. She climbed up. She sat down.

No pressure.
No prompting.
No urgency.

She didn't wee. She didn't poo. But she sat there chatting to me, calm and relaxed, talking about wee and poo like it was just part of life.

A few weeks earlier, this would have felt impossible.

That moment told me everything I needed to know:

• Her body felt safe

• Her mind felt curious, not threatened

• The toilet was no longer something to avoid

She was progressing.

Just not in the loud, obvious ways people usually talk about.

Progress Is Coming Back

Many children take pauses in toilet learning.

They lose interest.

They resist.

They step away to rest or reset.

This is not failure.

Progress often looks like *returning*.

• Coming back to the toilet after days or weeks of refusing

• Talking about it again after avoiding it

- Sitting again after illness, travel, or big emotions
- Trying once more after a regression

Coming back takes courage.

It means your child remembered safety.
They remembered trust.
They remembered this was a place they're allowed to learn.

Every return is a sign of resilience growing.

Progress isn't about never pausing.
It's about knowing it's safe to come back.

Celebrate the Tiny Wins – They Add Up

Write them down.
Say them loud.
Let yourself feel proud.

Because those tiny wins?
They are everything.

The first relaxed sit.
The calm after an accident.

The curiosity instead of fear.

The moment you feel a quiet something is shifting.

Those little wins make all the difference.

They soften the body.

They build trust.

They create safety.

And that safety is what eventually allows the wee and poo to happen in the toilet – not force, not pressure, not pushing through.

One day, often without warning, you'll look back and realise:

All those tiny moments were the progress.

They weren't delays.

They weren't detours.

They were the path.

Your child didn't just learn to use the toilet. They learned trust. Confidence. Safety. And you taught them that who they are, exactly as they are, is enough.

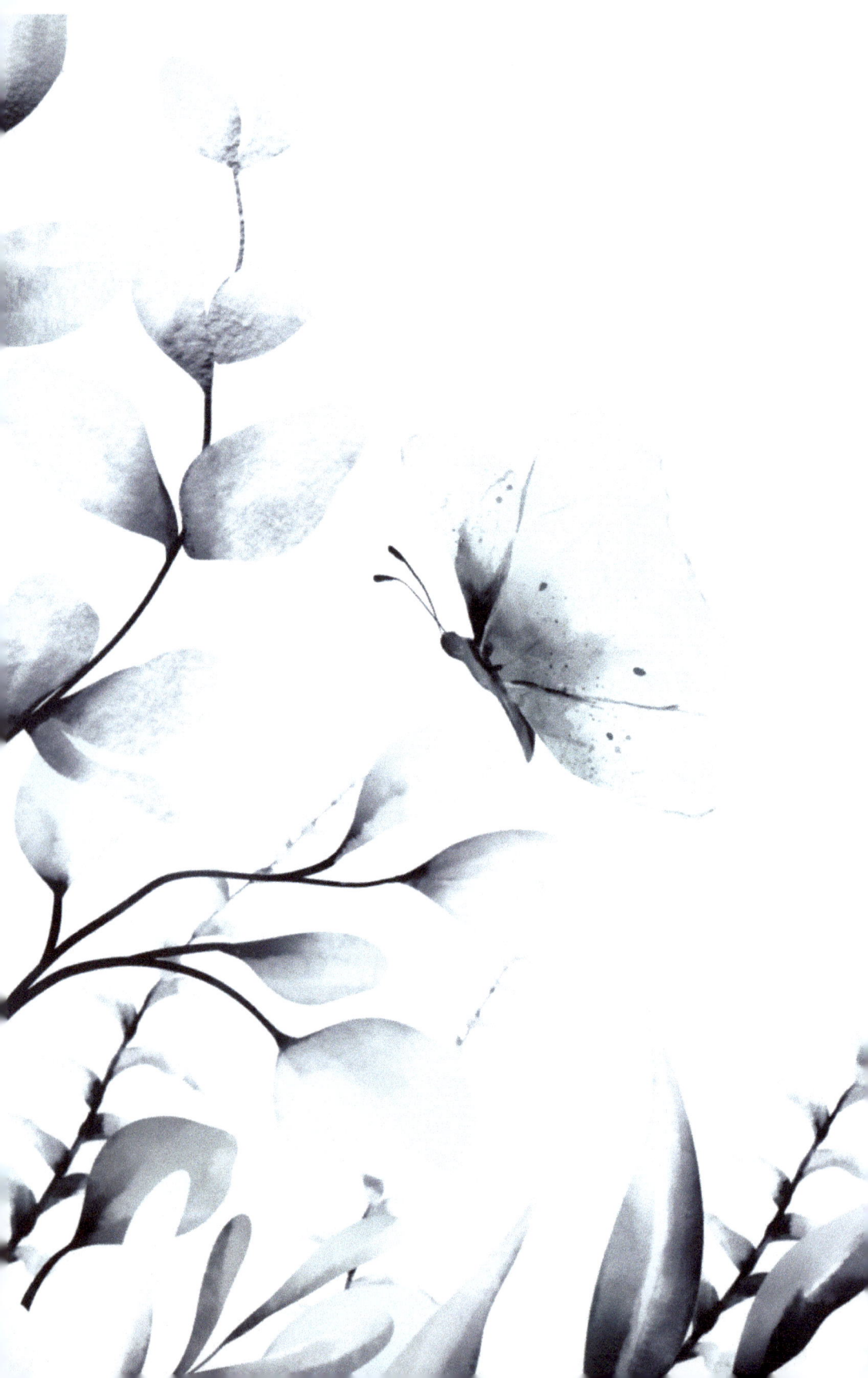

CHAPTER 9

Gentle Structure That Supports Safety

Toilet learning doesn't happen because we remind our child often enough. It happens when a child feels safe enough to listen to their body — and when the adults around them feel steady enough to slow down.

By this point in the book, you've already built the most important foundation: connection, trust, and emotional safety.

This chapter is about adding gentle structure to that foundation — not to control the process, but to support it.

Structure isn't pressure. When it's done well, it creates more ease.

<u>Why Gentle Structure Helps</u>

For many children — especially sensitive, late-talking, or neurodivergent children — uncertainty is harder than learning itself.

When a child doesn't know what will happen, how long it will last, or what's expected, their nervous system often tightens.

Gentle routines and predictable rhythms help a child relax, because nothing is a surprise.

Everything in this chapter is optional.

Take what helps.
Leave what doesn't.

Some families also find that simple visual supports — like picture cues or routine cards — can be helpful in toilet learning, especially for children who understand best through seeing rather than listening. These are optional tools, not a requirement.

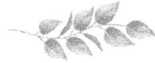

Part One: A Grounding Checklist

Before adding routines, it helps to pause. Not to prepare perfectly — but to notice what support is already in place.

Child Readiness (Emotional, Not Just Physical)

☐ Curious about the toilet or bathroom

☐ Comfortable being naked or semi-naked

☐ Able to pause briefly during play

☐ Accepts help with clothing

☐ Is soothed by your presence

☐ Communicates needs in any way

☐ Willing to sit — even briefly

They do not need all of these.

Readiness is not a checklist to complete.

It's a picture to notice.

Parent Readiness (This Matters Too)

☐ I understand accidents are part of learning

☐ I'm open to a slower timeline (often 2–12 weeks or longer)

☐ I can pause or adjust if things feel heavy

☐ I'm not tying outcomes to my worth as a parent

☐ I can stay calm even when nothing happens

If this list feels hard, it doesn't mean you can't do this.

It may simply mean you need more support.

Environment Check

☐ Toilet, potty, or both available

☐ Stable footing (step stool or floor support)

☐ Easy-to-remove clothing or bare-bottom time

☐ Wipes or toilet paper within reach

☐ Calm, familiar bathroom space

☐ Optional comfort items

The goal is access and ease — not perfection.

Part Two: A Gentle Daily Rhythm (Detailed)

This is not a strict schedule.

It's a flow you return to, day after day, with flexibility.

Morning: connection first, toilet offered once, optional sit, move on.

Mid-morning: quiet observation, gentle guidance if cues appear.

Before meals / leaving: offer, don't insist.

Afternoon: lower expectations, fewer words, more comfort.

Evening: wind down, no pushing, calm closure.

Part Three: When Less Is Better (Low-Word Routine)

Some children — and parents — need very little.

Morning

"The toilet is here."

Daytime

Watch quietly.

Guide if needed.

Clean up calmly.

Transitions

"Body check."

Evening

"We'll try again tomorrow."

That's enough.

A Simple Daytime Rhythm (At a Glance)

Some parents find it helpful to see what a gentle toileting day might look like.

This is not a schedule to follow closely.

It's simply a reference point — a way to picture the flow of the day.

Take what helps.

Leave the rest.

Morning

• Connection first (cuddles, calm start)

• Mention the toilet once: "The toilet is here if your body needs it."

• Optional sit if your child is willing

• Move on with the day

No pressure.

No expectation.

Mid-Morning / Playtime

• Bare-bottom time or easy clothing if possible

• Quiet observation

• Gentle support if cues appear

• Clean up calmly if accidents happen

This is often a natural learning window.

Before Lunch

• Offer, don't insist: "Before lunch, we can see if your body wants to try."

• Respect your child's answer.

Eating and regulation matter more than toileting outcomes.

After Lunch / Rest Time

• Lower expectations
• Short sits only, if any
• Comfort items welcome

Many children are tired here — accidents are common.

Nothing has gone wrong.

Afternoon

• Fewer reminders
• Familiar play
• Calm guidance if needed

Around day 3–4, many families find it helpful to:

• leave the house briefly
• go for a walk
• visit a familiar place

This can help your child's body learn that toileting is part of life — not something that only happens at home.

Keep outings short and low-pressure.

Before Dinner

• Gentle body check: "Before dinner, we can try if your body wants."
• No "last chance" language.

Evening

• Focus on winding down
• No pushing
• Acknowledge effort: "Your body is still learning."

End the day calm and connected.

Bedtime Reminder

Progress doesn't reset overnight.

What your child learns today stays with them — even if tomorrow looks different.

Part Four: Low-Pressure Days

Some days need to be lighter on purpose.

☐ Fewer reminders

☐ No timers

☐ No tracking outcomes

☐ Focus on connection

☐ Minimal language

☐ End the day regulated

Low-pressure days don't stop progress.

They support it.

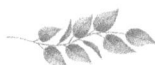

Closing This Section

Structure doesn't teach toileting.

Safety does.

Trust does.

Time does.

Everything in this section has been about what happens within the safety of your home — the place where your child can soften, settle, and keep learning in their own way.

There is no rush to finish this part.

No moment you have to force.

Learning will keep unfolding in small, sometimes invisible steps.

And when your child is ready for the next environment, you won't be starting over.

You'll be carrying what you've built with you — together.

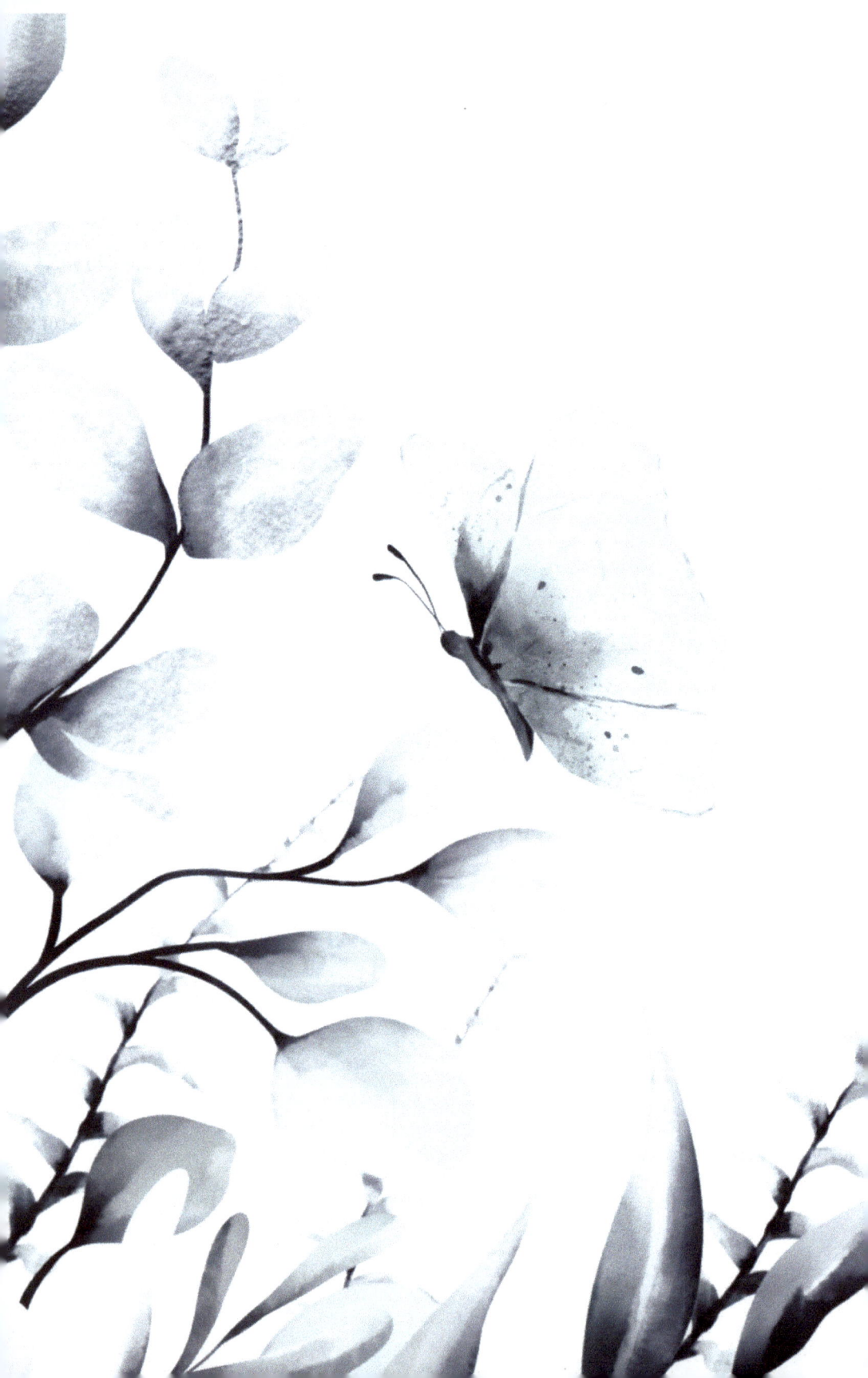

Chapter 10

Daycare, School & Big Transitions

How to Prepare, What's Normal, and Why It Can Feel Like Starting Again

D aycare or school is a huge emotional transition — not only for your child, but for you.

Even when your child knows the environment well, returning after toilet learning begins can feel like stepping into something entirely new. Toileting is no longer happening in the comfort of home. It's happening in unfamiliar bathrooms, with different sounds, smells, expectations, adults, and rhythms.

For many families, this brings uncertainty, emotional overload, and a sense that things have suddenly become harder.

This chapter is here to steady you. To help you understand what's happening beneath the surface, how to prepare gently, why progress can look different in this stage, and why much of the learning happening now is quiet — and meaningful.

The First Day Back After Toilet Learning

The first day back at daycare or school after toilet learning can feel tender — even if your child knows the environment well.

For your child, it's a new toileting world. Different bathrooms. Different routines. Different adults helping with something very personal. A lot to take in.

For you, it may feel like a small letting go. You might notice a mix of emotions — relief, uncertainty, hope, worry — all sitting together. You may wonder how your child will manage. How accidents will be handled. Whether progress will hold. Or quietly hope that being in a new space will help things feel easier.

These feelings don't mean you're unsure. They don't mean you've done anything wrong. They simply mean you care — and you're supporting your child through something new.

How to Prepare for Daycare (and What to Pack)

Preparation isn't about control. It's about safety — for your child and for you.

Preparing Your Child Emotionally

Before daycare, your child benefits most from warmth, predictability, and simple language.

Keep conversations light and reassuring:

• "If your body needs a wee, you can go to the toilet at daycare too."
• "You can tell your teacher and they will help you."

Gentle morning rhythms can help anchor the day:

• "After breakfast, we'll try for a wee, then shoes, then daycare."

No lectures.
No pressure.
Just calm, familiar flow.

What to Pack

- 3–5 spare sets of clothes
- Underwear or training pants
- Wipes
- Wet bag
- Socks
- A comfort item

Some parents also find it helpful to include a short note for educators:

"We're using gentle reminders and soft language like 'Let's try for a wee.' No pressure needed."

Preparing Yourself

Expect accidents.

Expect tiredness.

Expect different rhythms.

Daycare isn't a setback.

It's a new environment for learning.

When Daycare Makes Everything Feel Hard Again

(Regression vs Adjustment)

After starting daycare or returning to school, you might notice changes that feel worrying:

• More accidents

• Refusal to sit

• Hiding or avoiding the toilet

• Increased clinginess

• Bigger emotional outbursts

When this happens, it can feel alarming. It's easy to wonder if something has gone wrong.

But this isn't a loss of skill.

What you're seeing is emotional overload — and adjustment.

Daycare asks a lot of your child's nervous system. They are managing noise, waiting, sharing, rules, transitions, sensory input, new adults, and time away from you.

All day, they work hard to hold themselves together.

When they come home — to the place where they feel safest — their body finally lets go.

That release can look like regression. But what's actually happening is adjustment.

Your child's brain and body are learning how to manage a bigger world.

Toilet learning doesn't disappear during this phase. It simply moves into the background while emotional energy is being used elsewhere. The skill is still there. It's just underneath everything they're processing.

As daycare becomes familiar and predictable, that energy often frees up again — and confidence returns quietly.

This isn't failure.
It's adjustment.

If this stage feels heavy, know that it doesn't require fixing — only time, safety, and trust.

What Parents Often Feel During Daycare Transitions

This stage can feel unexpectedly heavy for parents — especially around daycare.

You might feel anxious in the mornings, wondering how the day will go. You may replay drop-off in your mind, questioning whether you did or said the right thing. You might brace yourself at pick-up, unsure of what you'll hear.

Some days, you may feel relief when you're told your child was "fine." Other days, hearing about accidents or struggles can land harder than you expect — even when you know it's normal.

At home, things can feel just as complicated.

Your child may unravel in the afternoons or evenings. There may be more tears, more resistance, more emotional intensity. And you might find yourself wondering why everything feels harder here.

Often, the hardest part isn't the toileting itself. It's trying to stay patient and gentle when your own nervous system is tired too.

These feelings don't mean you're doing something wrong.

They mean you are navigating a big transition alongside your child.

You are not failing.

You are adjusting too.

And that deserves care.

Supporting Toilet Learning Through Daycare Transitions

(and Why Home Can Feel Harder)

During daycare transitions, softness matters more than progress.

This stage isn't about pushing skills forward. It's about supporting recovery.

After a full day of managing the outside world, many children need home to be a place where nothing is asked of them straight away.

At home, gentle support often looks like:

• Lowering expectations
• Increasing cuddles and physical closeness
• Allowing decompression time before toilet reminders
• Choosing low-pressure days when needed
• Keeping routines predictable
• Praising effort and willingness, not outcomes

Helpful phrases can anchor safety first:

- "You're safe now."
- "It was a big day."
- "Your body worked so hard today."
- "Let's slow down for a bit."

If your child isn't weeing at home right now, there are many gentle reasons — and none of them are wrong.

Home is where you notice, and being noticed can sometimes feel like pressure.

Emotional transitions can make even soft attention feel big.

Some children save their body's "letting go" for school, where the emotional load is lighter.

Others are simply tired — especially around weeks two to three, when motivation often dips.

This phase is very common.

You're not restarting toilet learning.

You're supporting emotional recovery.

When Willingness Shows Up at School First

What you're seeing isn't refusal.
And it isn't failure.

It's your child responding differently to different environments.

For many sensitive, observant children, school or daycare can feel easier for practising new skills.

There is structure.
A predictable rhythm.
Other children modelling the behaviour.
Less emotional weight tied to each attempt.

At home, your child relaxes.

Home is where the guard comes down.
Where emotions are released.
Where effort pauses.

So it's not unusual for willingness to appear first at school — and resistance to show up at home.

That difference doesn't mean your child is confused.

It means they are regulating in the way that feels safest to them.

Little releases at school matter more than they appear to.

They are small, quiet signs that something is unfolding beneath the surface.

That your child's body is beginning to trust the process.

That muscles are starting to coordinate.

That the nervous system is allowing a gentle opening — even if it's brief, even if it's slow.

In this stage, what can look like "little wee drops" are actually meaningful milestones — early signs that trust, timing, and release are beginning to come together.

For many children, progress arrives this way.

Quietly.
In fragments.

Your child knows what to do.

They are simply practising where it feels easiest right now.

And that choice is part of learning.

Educator-Facing Support Box (Optional)

Some parents find it helpful to share a short note like this with educators. This is simply an example — take what feels right, change the wording, or leave it entirely.

For Educators: Supporting Toilet Learning Gently

This child is in the early stages of toilet learning. A calm, supportive approach helps them feel safe and confident as they practise.

Emotional safety, gentle language, and predictable routines tend to support success more than pressure.

Accidents are expected during this stage and are a normal part of learning.

Helpful approaches may include:

• Gentle reminders offered calmly (around every 45–60 minutes)

• Soft, neutral language such as "Let's try for a wee," or "Your body can take its time"

• Allowing the child to sit without expectation

• Supporting independence where possible, at the child's pace

It can help to avoid:

• Rushing or creating urgency

• Using rewards or consequences around toileting

• Showing disappointment after accidents

When home and daycare work together with consistency and kindness, children often feel safe enough to practise and progress naturally.

A Gentle Reminder for You

If daycare makes everything feel hard again, remember:

You didn't lose progress.

Your child didn't forget.

Your work wasn't undone.

Your child is learning how to hold a bigger world.

And you are still their anchor.

You are not failing.

You are loving them through one of the biggest transitions of their little life.

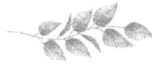

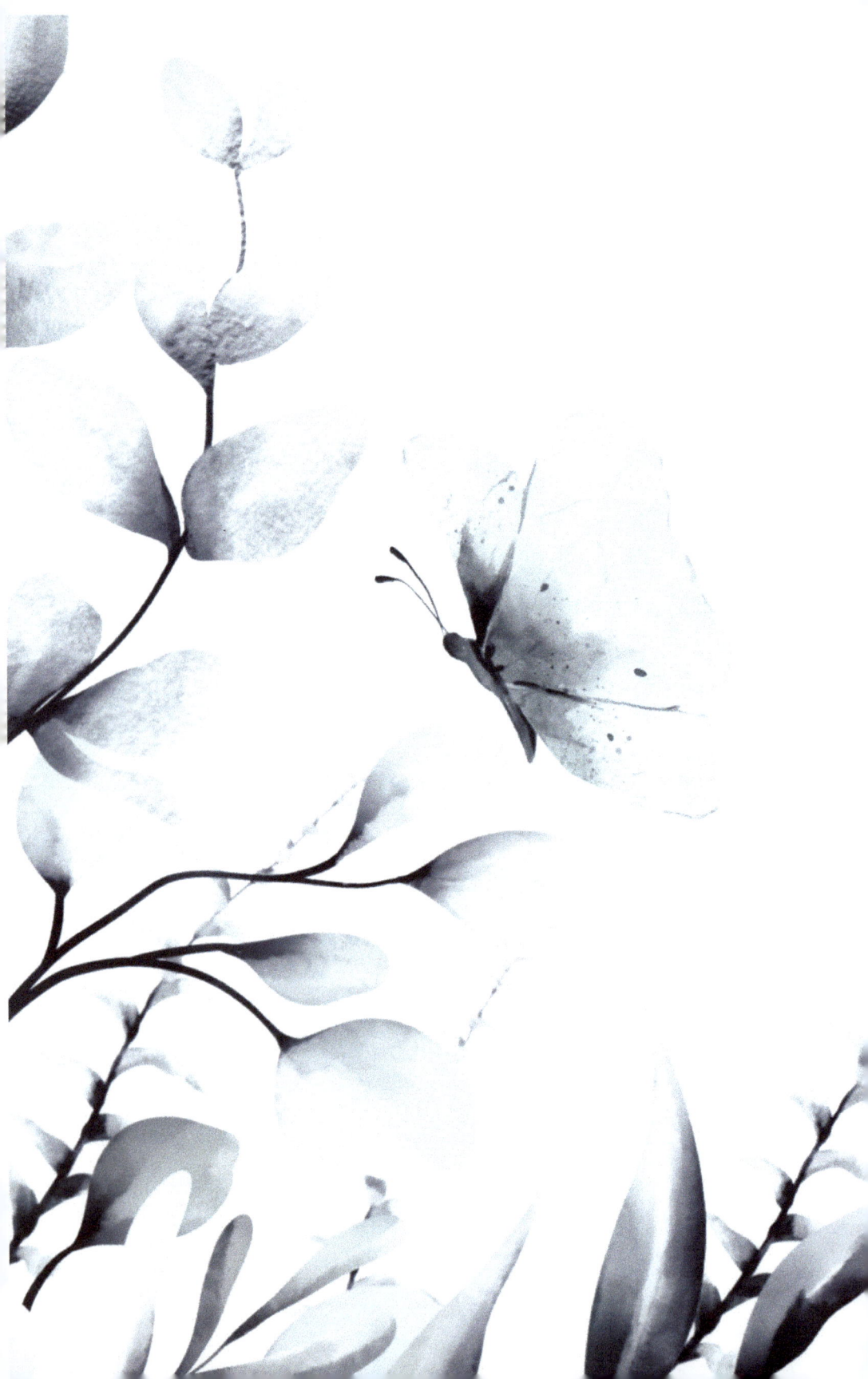

FINAL CHAPTER
YOU'RE NOT ALONE

One day, this season will quietly pass.

The nappies will be gone.

The spare clothes won't be packed anymore.

The bathroom routines will become simple and ordinary.

And what will remain will not be:

• how long it took
• how many accidents there were
• which method you followed

What will remain is how your child felt while learning.

Your child's body will remember:

• that they were never rushed
• that mistakes were met with safety

- that their signals were listened to
- that fear was met with softness
- that learning felt gentle
- that they were allowed to go at their own pace

They will carry forward:

"My body is safe."

"I am safe to try."

"I am safe to fail."

"I am safe to grow."

You didn't just teach your child where wee and poo go.

You taught them:

- how to listen to their body
- how to regulate through discomfort
- how to trust support
- how to move through fear
- how to try again without shame

This journey was never only about toilet learning.

It was always about relationship.

There were moments of joy too — quiet ones, unexpected ones.

A proud look.

A small success.

A laugh in the bathroom.

A day that felt lighter.

Those moments didn't erase the hard ones.

And the hard ones didn't undo the good.

They were all part of the same learning.

If you ever doubted yourself...

If you ever cried quietly after a hard day...

If you ever wondered if you were doing damage instead of doing good...

You did not break your child.

You protected them.

You held them.

You led with love — even when you were tired.

If you are still in the thick of it:

You are not behind.

You are not doing this wrong.

You are building something that cannot be rushed.

Every cuddle after an accident.

Every quiet redirect.

Every soft "It's okay."

Every low-pressure day.

Every time you chose connection instead of control.

It all counted.

Toilet learning from the inside out was never about quick results.

It was always about:

• safety before skill

• regulation before release

• trust before independence

• connection before correction

And you honoured that.

This book was never meant to deliver an outcome. It was meant to hold you steady while your child found their own.

You didn't create the outcome. You created the safety that allowed it to arrive.

If this book has given you softer expectations, stronger trust in your child, or deeper trust in yourself, then it has done its job.

You were never meant to do this alone.

With heart,

Elise Hansford

www.ingramcontent.com/pod-product-compliance
Lightning Source LLC
Chambersburg PA
CBHW052012030426

42334CB00029BA/3183